LIBERATION

An IFS-inspired companion for psychedelic and ancestral medicine experiences

TASHA HUNTER
MSW, LCSW

Copyright © 2024 by Tasha Hunter

All rights reserved. No part of this book may be reproduced or used in any manner without written permission of the copyright owner except for the use of quotations in a book review.

FIRST EDITION Printed in the United States of America

www.tashahunterlcsw.com

Paperback: ISBN 978-1-7344178-0-7

Tasha Hunter's books may be purchased for educational, business, or sales and promotional use. For information, please email the author at tashahunterauthor@gmail.com.

Library of Congress Control Number: 2024920138

Cover Design: Tasha Hunter and Jana Rade

Interior Layout: Tasha Hunter and Jana Rade

Published in association with Aheri Press

This journal belongs to:

_____

"When we practice loving ourselves, we, in turn, learn to love others in a more healthy and balanced way."

~TASHA HUNTER

Disclaimer

This journal is ideal for processing and tracking psychedelic and ancestral medicine experiences, trips, and ceremonies. The content is for informational and personal reflections only. It does not endorse or promote the use of illegal substances, nor does it serve as a substitute for professional, medical, or mental health treatment.

Please consult with a licensed healthcare provider before making any decisions related to drug use or therapy. The author encourages all readers to adhere to the laws and regulations of their respective jurisdictions. Psychedelic and ancestral medicine experiences should only occur in safe settings. The author does not promise any results of integration based on this workbook.

A Blessing:

May we honor our ancestors, both past and present.
May we honor all plant and animal beings.
May we honor our connection to nature and community.
May we honor (our own) *and* each other's backgrounds, traditions, identities, and cultures.

May we prioritize safety, consent, and bounda0art.
May we listen without interrupting or dismissing our parts.

May we honor privacy and confidentiality in all healing settings.
May we have the courage to lay our burdens down and replace them with gifts.
May we heal and be liberated *together*.
May we remember that we belong to each other.

SACRED OFFERINGS

1. Sacred Offerings 5
2. Definitions 9
3. How Liberation Restores 11
4. Addressing Oppression in Psychedelic Spaces 13
5. Community Agreements 17
6. Establishing Workable Agreements 19
7. Repairing Rupture 23
8. Considerations For Psychedelic or Entheogenic Medicine Usage 25
9. Intention Setting 27
10. The Importance of Integration 29
11. In Pursuit Of Safety 31
12. Examples of Harm in Medicine Spaces 33
13. Questions to Ask the Medicine Facilitator 35
14. Pre-Integration Conversations Topics 36
15. Self-Qualities 39
16. Guided Journaling Worksheets ✎ 43
17. Journaling Pages ✎ 50
18. Parts Mapping Worksheets ✎ 51
19. Rituals ✎ 127
20. Four-Week Microdosing Trackers ✎ 131
21. Self- Energy Assessments ✎ 157
22. Letter to Your Younger Self ✎ 174
23. Letter to Your Parts ✎ 176
24. What are the Parts? 179
25. Resources 185
26. About the Author 187
27. Other Books 188
28. Heartfelt Appreciation 189

Sections marked with ✎ include additional journaling pages.

"We are not responsible for our oppression, but we must be responsible for our own liberation."

~MALCOLM X

Dear Fellow Seeker,

Welcome to the journey of healing. May this guided journal be your trusted companion and a safe space where your inner parts can be honored. This journal is an invitation to deepen the connection with yourself, reflect on your medicine experiences, and gently integrate the insights you uncover along the way. As you embark on this path, remember that every step — no matter how small — will lead you toward greater wholeness, healing, and liberation.

Here are a few instructions for using this guided companion:

Begin by grounding yourself in your purpose and reflect on what you hope to gain or heal through your therapeutic work and medicine experiences.

1. Create a sacred space where you feel safe and connected to yourself. Doing so might mean playing soothing music, lighting candles, or taking time to exhale. Let the space become a container where all of your parts feel welcomed.
2. A core tenet of Internal Family Systems (IFS) therapy is understanding our different parts (e.g., Managers, Firefighters, Exiles). You can use this journal to map, track, and communicate with your parts. Take the time to explore their needs, fears, roles, and stories.
3. For psychedelic and ancestral medicine sessions, this journal includes dedicated space to document dosage, setting, somatic responses, and any insights you experience on this journey. This tracking will help you integrate your medicine experiences with clarity and compassion.
4. Within this journal, you will find writing prompts. Take advantage of this space to process triggers, reactions, memories, and wisdom that your parts share.
5. Use this journal to track any changes to your internal system. Over time, I hope you will notice a deepening connection with your parts and how much you have become aligned and aware of your core Self.
6. For mental health professionals, coaches, and medicine facilitators, this guide will support your integration sessions.
7. This journal also includes conversation prompts and harm-reduction tips to encourage safer psychedelic and ancestral medicine experiences.
8. Above all, remember to approach this work with gentleness and much grace. Hold space for all the parts of yourself that yearn to be witnessed. Healing is *not* linear, and it is okay to feel however you feel at any moment.

With deep respect for your journey,

Tasha Hunter

"To be truly liberated, we must confront the parts of ourselves that are in hidden alliance with the systems that seek to destroy us."

~COLE ARTHUR RILEY

DEFINITIONS

1. **Ancestral Medicine or Entheogens:** include psychoactive plants or fungi used ceremonially or recreationally by indigenous communities. Examples include: cannabis, Psilocybin, Ayahuasca, Peyote, and Iboga.

2. **Exile/Wounded One:** parts that carry pain, shame, negative beliefs, energies, and burdens from trauma. They are often hidden and suppressed to prevent the person from feeling overwhelmed by the emotions.

3. **Facilitator:** a person who guides or supports a person through the medicine experience.

4. **Firefighter/Reactive Part:** a part that steps in when the wounded one's pain breaks through, attempting to distract or numb the person through impulsive, disassociative, or destructive behaviors.

5. **Integration:** understanding, processing, and incorporating emotions and experiences from a medicine experience.

6. **Burdens:** extreme energies, emotions/feelings, messages, beliefs, practices, coping strategies, and conditioning that is carried in the system.

Examples:
- **Ancestral burden:** family patterns, illness, mental health issues, religious/spiritual beliefs, gender and identity beliefs.
- **Cultural burden:** racism, oppression, homophobia, transphobia, ageism, sexism, sizeism, ableism, and colorism.
- **Global burden:** colonization, food insecurities, health disparities, poverty, LGBTQIA rights, climate change, pandemics, and war.
- **Legacy burden:** any belief, emotion, coping mechanism, behavior, or practice that is passed down intergenerationally - slavery, povery, addiction, anger, hyperindependence.
- **Personal burden:** abuse, neglect, microaggressions, violence, any painful pre-traumatic memory or experience.

7. **Manager/Proactive Part:** a part that tries to keep the person safe by managing day-to-day life, controlling behaviors, and avoiding behaviors that might trigger the Exile/Wounded One.

8. **Parts:** various subpersonalities or aspects of a person's psyche, each with its own perspective, feelings, and roles.

9. **Post-Integration:** a process that follows the medicine experience that involves making changes, embodying lessons, and sustaining lessons long-term.

10. **Pre-Integration:** the preparatory phase before a medicine experience. Discussion about the scene, setting, safety, intentions, and supportive resources will occur.

11. **Psychedelics:** powerful psychoactive substances that alter perception and mood and can affect cognitive processes. Examples include MDMA, LSD, DMT, and Ketamine.

12. **Queerness:** a critical engagement that challenges traditional norms and values by challenging and deconstructing binary thinking and mainstream societal expectations and values, particularly relating to cis-hetero patriarchies.

13. **Self:** a person's core or authentic self that is not impacted by traumatic experiences. The goal of IFS is to develop a relationship between the self and parts.

14. **Trip Sitter:** a person who provides support and supervision during the medicine experience.

15. **Unburdening:** a process in IFS that helps a part(s) to release burdensome thoughts, feelings/emotions, behaviors, beliefs, or responsibilites.

HOW LIBERATION RESTORES

Liberation is an IFS-inspired companion designed to support you on your path toward personal growth and healing. This journal is informed by an intersectional, inclusive, and harm-reduction approach. Whether you are using psychedelics or ancestral medicine spiritually, recreationally, or therapeutically, I created this guide to accompany you on your transformative journey and to promote safer medicine experiences. This companion will be your space holder as you:

1. Understand internalized oppression such as racism, sexism, homophobia, transphobia, patriarchy, and capitalism, which lead to harmful beliefs about oneself and others.
2. Address and challenge internalized oppression, recognizing its impact on self-esteem, self-worth, and survival.
3. Address the wounds of systemic violence and historical traumas, reducing the impact on your daily life.
4. For people who benefit from systems of privilege (e.g., white people in white supremacy culture), this IFS-inspired companion can assist with exploring parts that hold internalized dominance and xenophobia. This includes parts that feel entitled, fearful of loss of power/privilege/control, dismissive or defensive parts, or those that hold implicit bias.
5. Allow access to wounded, abused, and abandoned parts that carry painful memories, shame, perfectionism, distrust, hyper-independence, and other burdens.
6. Uncover and unburden global, ancestral, cultural, and personal legacy burdens.
7. Reduce the impact of hypervigilant and defensive parts that make wholeness more difficult to access in non-altered states. Psychedelics and ancestral medicines often allow greater access to self-energy.
8. Amplify and access self-energy (i.e., compassion, clarity, curiosity, courage, etc.), which will make it easier to build a relationship with wounded Exiles and to (better) understand the proactive and reactive responses of Managers and Firefighters.
9. Promote a deeper emotional awareness and clarity regarding parts' roles, who they protect, and the fears and concerns that have kept them in their roles.
10. Set intentions and self-reflect to help you navigate past and present challenges.
11. Practice self-compassion by acknowledging and validating your experiences, history, emotions, and needs.

12. Understand and reflect on the various aspects of your identity and how they intersect, recognizing the unique strengths and challenges they may bring. Explore ways to embrace your authentic self and express your identity.
13. Support yourself as you engage in activities that allow you to celebrate the fullness of your authenticity, culture, and diversity.
14. Explore and incorporate other healing strategies such as mindfulness, breathing, rest, creative outlets, and inclusion within a safe and supportive community.
15. Prioritize harm-reduction practices for substance use, including strategies for safer consumption, overdose prevention, integration, aftercare, and supportive services.
16. Reduce the stigma associated with psychedelics and ancestral medicine, which will increase access and make them safer for all.
17. When IFS therapy/coaching aligns with psychedelics and ancestral medicine, it can accelerate the healing process and lead to more embodied self-love and self-compassion.

ADDRESSING OPPRESSION IN PSYCHEDELIC SPACES

Beloved, it's time to face the hard truths about the spaces we step into. We need to name the fear, the fragility, and the barriers to truth-telling around oppression and racism in these healing spaces, especially in psychedelics and ancestral medicine. Silence and neutrality create fear-based, unsafe spaces. Too often, we're met with a lack of safety where the roots of this medicine—its Indigenous history and its sacredness—are ignored or disrespected. We need to address these issues boldly, vocally, on social media, and in our policies. Justice must be present in all aspects of our work…in advocacy, therapy, and spiritual care, too.

If you're a person of color, especially Black, I know this journey carries a particular weight for you. There's the constant question: Will this be a space that truly sees me, holds me, and respects the entirety of who I am? Will this be a space that acknowledges and takes accountability for harm?

To those leading and creating these spaces—this is a call to face your own fear and fragility. Go beyond performative allyship. Doing the work means you need to get uncomfortable. It means recognizing and learning about the very real, very deep wounds of racism, colonization, and appropriation. Center the voices of the marginalized and ensure that your spaces are built with inclusivity and respect at their core.

Here's what we need to do together:

Silence and neutrality have no place in healing: Explicitly address racism and oppression in your words, policies, and every area of practice.

Build genuine relationships with Black, Brown, and Indigenous communities: This means consistent engagement and true accountability.

Honor Indigenous traditions, spirituality, and healing practices: Approach this work with respect and acknowledge the deep roots of these practices.

Create programs that elevate marginalized voices: Structure training and organizational frameworks that lift up Black, Brown, and Indigenous healers, women scholars, and leaders, including medicine facilitators and subject matter experts.

Provide diverse resources for clients: Include multicultural books, research, peer-reviewed articles, art, and music to enrich the healing journey.

Foster belonging intentionally: Make room for all identities, particularly Black, Brown, Indigenous, women, and LGBTQIA. Go beyond mere inclusivity—actively cultivate spaces where everyone feels a profound sense of belonging.

Welcome lived experiences without threat: Invite people from underrepresented groups to share their stories, free from denial, spiritual bypassing, weaponization of mental health language, or invalidation.

Give back with accountability: Establish reciprocal practices with Indigenous communities, and share these practices publicly to hold yourself accountable.

Make services accessible through anti-oppressive fee structures: Implement sliding scale options, scholarships, and pro bono services to ensure therapy, coaching, medicine facilitation, and training are accessible to everyone, especially those affected by systemic oppression.

Cultivate safety and inclusion as non-negotiable standards: Every employee, volunteer, intern, and client should actively commit to creating a safe, inclusive environment, particularly for those with less power and privilege. This includes steadfast support for LGBTQIA individuals, women, people with disabilities, Black, Brown, and Indigenous communities. Everyone must embody respect, empathy, and a dedication to equity, knowing their role is essential in ensuring all voices are valued and protected.

Let's stand in bravery together. This is the season for uncompromised truth. May we demand and create spaces that are not just safe but deeply committed to anti-oppression and respect for all of us, especially those who've been silenced for far too long.

BRAVE SPACES
(ORIGINALLY INSPIRED BY BETH STRANO'S POEM BELOW)

Together we will create brave space
because there is no such thing as a "safe space" — We exist in the real world.
We all carry scars and we have all caused wounds.
In this space
We seek to turn down the volume of the outside world,
We amplify voices that fight to be heard elsewhere,
We call each other to more truth and love
We have the right to start somewhere and continue to grow.
We have the responsibility to examine what we think we know.
We will not be perfect.
This space will not be perfect.
It will not always be what we wish it to be
But It will be our brave space together, and
We will work on it side by side.

—Mickey ScottBey Jones

There is no such thing as a "safe space"—
We exist in the real world.
We all carry scars and have caused wounds.
This space
seeks to turn down the volume of the world outside,
and amplify voices that have to fight to be heard elsewhere,
This space will not be perfect.
It will not always be what we wish it to be
But
It will be our space together,
and we will work on it side by side.

—Beth Strano

"Now is when you root deeper into your holy things. Be a living ceremony."

~JAIYA JOHN

COMMUNITY AGREEMENTS

- Come with open hearts and open minds. Lead with kindness, compassion, and respect toward yourself and others.
- Honor the plants, animals, fungi, and humans involved in this healing work.
- Listen, learn, and advocate for people from underrepresented or marginalized communities.
- Look out for one another. If someone is at risk of harm or danger, speak up, offer help, or seek support.
- Avoid making assumptions about another person's intentions, identity, or motives, including their orientation or the pronunciation of their name.
- Respect boundaries. Seek permission before offering feedback or touching another person.
- Respect and listen to your inner parts. Know that you have the choice of what to share and what to keep private.
- Speak from your own experience. Use "I" statements rather than "we."
- Be mindful of the space you make and take when in the presence of others.
- Commit to confidentiality. Share the wisdom gained here, but leave out any identifying details and experiences of others unless you have permission.
- All parts are welcome, but not all behaviors. No physical or verbal harm to self or others.
- Be open to hard conversations and practice witnessing the parts that may want to avoid conflict.
- When speaking, be mindful of intent versus impact. Regardless of your intention, take responsibility for the impact of your words and actions on others.
- Sit with discomfort. If you've harmed someone, listen to them rather than defend.
- Create space for multiple truths and norms. Speak your truth and seek understanding of truths that differ from yours, with awareness of power dynamics.
- If your system becomes triggered by another person's share, practice acknowledging your activated parts. If you need extra support, feel free to ask.

- Strong emotions are natural and common here. Vulnerability can activate protective parts. Trust in your ability to care for any parts needing quiet, grounding, a break, or sustenance.
- If your learning needs differ from what is being offered, please let us know so we can ensure you're getting what you need.
- There may be times when the group leader needs to interrupt. This is non-negotiable; however, we can decide together how you would like to be interrupted.

ESTABLISHING WORKABLE AGREEMENTS

In Internal Family Systems (IFS) therapy, "contracting" or "workable agreements" (both terms used interchangeably) is a foundational process that establishes safety, autonomy, and trust between the practitioner and the client. In psychedelic-assisted therapy and ancestral medicine settings, this process becomes even more critical, as expanded states of consciousness can heighten vulnerability, surface deeply held trauma, and bring forth unexpected inner dynamics. To create workable agreements, a flexible, anti-oppressive, and consent-based approach is necessary. **Empowerment and agency are everything in this process.** Before beginning deep inner work, it is essential to:

- Establish **Self-to-part relationships** to build internal trust and safety.
- Identify **protectors who may hold fear, shame, doubt, or resistance** to the process.
- Acknowledge **cultural, ancestral, and systemic burdens** that may impact parts' willingness to engage.
- Ensure **ongoing consent** from **both the client and their parts**, recognizing that agreements may need adjustment over time.

KEY QUESTIONS FOR INITIAL PART CHECK-INS:

- "How does your system feel about entering this process?"
- "Are there any protectors that have concerns about what might happen?"
- "Do you sense any fear, skepticism, or resistance from certain parts?"
- "How can we ensure all parts feel safe and included in this work?"
- "How do your parts feel about adding medicine to your healing work?"

Many clients, particularly those from the Global Majority and LGBTQIA+ communities, have parts that may resist engaging due to fears of:

- **Being overpowered, controlled, or unheard** by the therapist.
- **Re-traumatization** through unconscious replication of colonial or oppressive dynamics.
- The **medicine experience itself** feeling scary or overwhelming.
- Worries about potential **legal consequences**.

- Concerns about facing **criticism** from others.
- Anxiety about **personal information or secrets being exposed**.
- Apprehension about **experiencing health crises**.
- **The stigma** associated with using psychedelic and ancestral medicines for healing.
- **Revealing deep wounds.**
- Feel **shame** about needing healing or appearing "broken."
- Carry **internalized oppression** (e.g., a critic part reinforcing survival beliefs from white supremacy, patriarchy, or ableism).
- Experience **dissociation, fragmentation, or shutdown** when thinking about inner work.
- **"Doing it wrong"** or unintentionally **harming an exile**.
- Worry about **forming dependence on the therapist, space holder, or medicine**.

HOW TO ADDRESS THESE PARTS COMPASSIONATELY:

- **"You and your system are in charge. We move at your pace."**
- "If any part is not ready, we **pause** and listen to its concerns."
- "We will **periodically revisit** our workable agreements to honor shifts in your internal system."
- "You have the right to **opt out, modify, or withdraw** from any practice at any time."
- "I'd love to hear what concerns this part has about going inside."
- "If a part is scared —we don't force anything."
- "We will **work with protectors first**, before going to exiles."
- "Your system will always show us what it's ready for—**we trust its timing**."

Flexibility is key. Remember, **IFS-informed work is not linear**—parts may shift their willingness at different stages, requiring continual re-evaluation of agreements.

WORKABLE AGREEMENT STATEMENTS FOR MEDICI NE EXPERIENCES

- "Would you like a grounding touch, a weighted blanket, or a verbal check-in if things feel too intense?"
- "If a protector shows up, **they do not have to step aside**. We will respect them and we will listen."
- "Some parts may suddenly **feel unsafe, skeptical, or disconnected**—that's okay. We will honor them."
- "If unexpected emotions or ancestral burdens arise, **we take it slow**."
- "Although you may feel alone, I am here to remind you that you are safe and supported."

After the medicine experience, parts may **shift perspectives, feel unsettled, or resist integration**. Re-contracting in this phase is key:

REASSESSING READINESS:

- "How do your parts feel about what came up?"
- "Are there any that feel unsettled, scared, or regretful?"
- "Some parts may resist 'going back to normal'—that's okay."
- "Let's set agreements for gentle integration, allowing space for reflection, ritual, or rest."
- "This is an ongoing conversation—your system will keep telling us what it needs."

THERAPIST/PRACTITIONER SELF-WORK

The therapist must also engage in **their own inner work** to ensure:

- They are **not unconsciously reinforcing oppressive dynamics** (e.g., being an authority over the client's system).
- They can **hold their own parts** that may get activated in the process.
- They recognize **when a client needs more agency, less structure, or different pacing**.
- They check their **own biases** around what "successful" or "right" healing looks like.

SAMPLE IFS CONTRACT FOR PSYCHEDELIC/ANCESTRAL HEALING

"In this process, you and your system are in charge. We will engage with your inner world at a pace that feels safe and honoring to all parts of you. I will listen for concerns from any protectors who may feel hesitant, skeptical, or afraid of this work. We will check in regularly to ensure that agreements still feel aligned and adjust them as needed."

"During the medicine journey, you have full autonomy over your experience. If any part becomes overwhelmed, uncertain, or needs a break, we will pause and listen. You do not need to force anything or go deeper than what feels right. I trust your system's timing, and I will support you in navigating this process with care and respect."

"After the journey, we will integrate what arose in a way that supports your ongoing healing. Some parts may feel differently after the experience, and that's okay. We will take our time, adjusting as needed. Your healing process is yours, and I am here to support you in whatever way feels most aligned."

ADDRESSING POTENTIAL RUPTURES IN THE THERAPEUTIC ALLIANCE

In any therapeutic relationship, especially within the context of IFS and psychedelic or ancestral medicine work, it's essential to acknowledge the possibility of misunderstandings or tensions—commonly referred to as "ruptures." Proactively discussing how to handle such situations during the contracting phase fosters trust and safety. This openness requires courage from both the client and the practitioner and underscores the collaborative nature of the therapeutic journey.

Strategies for Addressing Ruptures:

- **Normalize the Possibility:** Acknowledge that disagreements or misunderstandings can occur and are a natural part of the therapeutic process.
- **Establish Open Communication:** Encourage clients to voice any discomfort or concerns as they arise, ensuring they feel heard and valued.
- **Collaborative Problem-Solving:** Work together to understand the root of the rupture and develop strategies to repair and strengthen the therapeutic alliance.

By integrating these practices into the initial contracting phase, both client and practitioner commit to a transparent therapeutic relationship, enhancing the potential for healing and growth.

REPAIRING RUPTURE

1. Acknowledge that harm or abuse has occurred and that this painful or traumatic experience impacts both individuals and their relationship. Recognize that the harm may also affect others in the community.
2. Engage with any parts of yourself that may feel confused, hurt, guilty, ashamed, embarrassed, or responsible. Allow all parts to be present.
3. Respect the right of the harmed person to experience and express their feelings, addressing their wounds without interference from protective parts like denial or justification.
4. With curiosity, honesty, and compassion for yourself and the injured party, identify the parts within you that may feel activated.
5. Take a deep breath. Let your parts know that you're aware of their presence.
6. Listen to the perspectives of these parts without letting them dominate or minimize the harm caused.
7. Ask your parts to step back slightly or hold space so that you can be fully present with the situation.
8. Extend an honest apology that clearly names the harm caused, centering the person affected by the injury.
9. Remain open and present as you listen to the other person's pain. Stay with your own discomfort as you witness their anger, sadness, distrust, or other strong emotions.
10. Recognize and name systemic and historical factors that may amplify the impact of the harm.
11. Work together to determine what meaningful reparation could look like. This may include:
    - A physical gesture (like a hug)
    - Words of affirmation or validation
    - Naming boundary and safety violations
    - Public acknowledgment of wrongdoing
    - Disrupting and addressing cult-like or oppressive community behaviors (e.g., siding with the abuser, blaming the victim, character assassination, or shunning)
    - Financial compensation
    - Diversity, Equity, and Inclusion (DEI) consultation
    - Intentional steps to prevent future harm
    - Actions to rebuild a healthy relationship
    - Stepping down from a platform or position of power

12. Agree to check in with the other person as often as needed or as mutually agreed.
13. Reinforce your dedication to personal accountability, healing, safety, and ethical behavior.
14. Learning how to repair is an ongoing practice—we may not get it right the first time, but it's important to keep trying.

CONSIDERATIONS FOR PSYCHEDELIC OR ENTHEOGENIC MEDICINE USAGE

Entering an altered state with psychedelics and ancestral medicines is not solely about love, peace, or beautiful imagery. While these experiences can bring profound insights, they may also evoke intense, unpredictable responses that can be physically, emotionally, and spiritually challenging. It can get real and be really scary all at the same time.

These powerful experiences affect both body and mind. You may encounter vivid imagery, unsettling or frightening sounds, uncontrollable crying or laughter, body tremors, muscle tension, temperature fluctuations, nausea, bowel disturbances, and changes in breathing or heart rate.

These physical reactions are natural but may feel intense or overwhelming. Beyond these immediate effects, psychedelic journeys often trigger:

Emotional Releases: The experience may unlock deeply held emotions, including sadness, fear, anger, rage, joy, euphoria, or relief. These feelings can arise suddenly, allowing for emotional catharsis and the potential for healing.

Spiritual Insights and Transformation: Psychedelics can open pathways to spiritual insights, creating a deepened connection to oneself, others, nature, or the universe. This can feel transformative, disorientating, or unstable.

Relationship and Social Dynamics: As old patterns and beliefs come into focus, shifts may emerge in how you relate to others. Psychedelics can reveal needs for healthier boundaries, desires for different relationship dynamics, or a new appreciation for meaningful, emotionally safe connections.

Impulses for Major Life Changes: During or after the experience, there may be a strong urge to make significant life changes— changing careers, relocating, starting a new career, or embracing new, wellness rituals. practices. While these insights can be profound, it's essential to approach them with discernment, patience, and a clear mind after the altered state has passed.

Such experiences can be life-changing but also destabilizing, making integration crucial. Processing these insights with trusted support or integration resources, including grounding practices, journaling, therapy, or community, can help bring clarity and stability, allowing for thoughtful and lasting growth.

INTENTION SETTING

Setting intentions is the first and most important step in creating meaningful change. It's a way to prioritize and focus on the next steps in your healing journey. According to an article on MindBloom.com, an intention can be:

An outcome you want to achieve
An experience you wish to have in the session
A request for insights or healing in specific areas of your life
A desire to see or develop certain characteristics within yourself
Take some time to think about what you hope to gain from this psychedelic or ancestral experience.

Examples:

"I want to have fun."
"I want to heal my grief and depression." "I want to connect with my ancestors."
"I want to understand myself better."
"I want the medicine to reveal what I need to know."

Check with Your Parts: See if any parts of you feel ambivalent, afraid, or uncertain about this healing path.

Choose 1-3 Intentions: Write them down. Discuss them with your therapist, coach, or medicine facilitator.

Practice Grounding: Use meditation or other grounding practices to help you center on your intentions before the medicine experience.

And Finally... Remember, if the experience feels intense, you can always tell your parts: "We signed up for healing, not an episode of Amazing Race!!"

Reference:
https://www.mindbloom.com/blog/your-complete-guide-to-setting-intentions

"Medicine is not a magical cure but a part of the process of healing."

CHRIS BURRIS

THE IMPORTANCE OF INTEGRATION

How many steps did you take to arrive at this point of choosing psychedelic or ancestral medicine as the next step in your healing? How many questions, plans, and decisions were involved? How much time, energy, and money did it require? This healing path is a privilege and, often, a sacrifice. And this is why integration is so crucial. It's a process, not a one-time event—and one that most of us know well from other life transitions. Think about the times you've explored changes in your mind and body, taken note of new awarenesses, discussed next steps, or tried to incorporate new routines and make plans for your future. That process? That's integration. It's the intentional act of taking the insights and shifts from a powerful experience—like one with psychedelics or ancestral medicine—and making them meaningful, useful, and lasting. For those of you seeking deep, long-term changes in your healing journey, this guide to integration is for you.

If the integrative process is new to you, know that it's been here long before us. Integration is deeply rooted and grounded in Indigenous culture—a sacred practice that honors the wisdom of experiences and is woven into the fabric of spiritual and communal healing. Indigenous cultures have always recognized the importance of taking what we learn, finding meaning, and integrating it into daily life. We honor these traditions and their immense contributions to healing practices today.

WHAT IS INTEGRATION?

Integration is everything that happens *after* a psychedelic or ancestral medicine experience, and it is one of the most important processes to support long-lasting change. The medicine experience brings you what you need, but integration is where you take those lessons, find meaning, and solidify real shifts. This process is essential, not something to ignore or push to the background. Integration allows us to ground insights, gain clarity, and build on the changes we want to make in our lives.

Many of us use integration with medicines like MDMA, Ayahuasca, Iboga, Cannabis, Ketamine, Psilocybin, and San Pedro. It's part of a broader healing practice that deserves as much care and intention as the medicine experience itself. This is why it should be discussed beforehand during what's known as the preparation stage, then revisited in the hours and days afterward as part of the integration process.

INTEGRATION AS A CONTINUOUS PROCESS

Integration isn't something that happens once. It's an ongoing, deeply personal ritual of mental, physical, emotional, and spiritual care. It requires regular attention, dedication, and the support of a safe structure. I suggest a three-pronged approach for integration that includes:

1. Community:

Engage in a safe group or supportive community that values this healing work.

2. Professional Guidance:

Work with a therapist, practitioner, coach, or spiritual leader who can guide and support you through the integration process.

3. Self-led Practices:

Cultivate your own self-led practices that support reflection, grounding, and growth.

Not everyone uses psychedelics or ancestral medicines as part of a therapeutic process or for long-term transformation. But for those of you who do, remember: integration is a choice. It's the bridge between insight and change, between experience and embodiment. Take it seriously, let it become part of your life.

For more on integration read: https://chacruna.net/expanded-access-to-the-art-of-integration/

IN PURSUIT OF SAFETY

Harm within psychedelic and ancestral medicine spaces is common and must be addressed. As a Black, queer, and cis-gendered woman, I am most concerned about psychedelics and ancestral medicine usage within historically marginalized and underrepresented communities. I am specifically speaking about harm reduction for Black and Brown People of Color, Women or female-identifying, and LGBTQIA+ communities. We must protect ourselves and each other for several important reasons:

1. Historical and Societal Factors

Throughout history, historically marginalized and underrepresented communities (i.e., Black, Brown, LGBTQIA+) have faced discrimination, oppression, and systemic disadvantages. These factors have resulted in a lack of representation, exclusion, limited resource access, and unequal power dynamics.

2. Safety and Well-being

Ancestral Medicine experiences can be deeply personal and emotionally intense. Creating a safe and supportive environment is essential for individuals to navigate these experiences effectively. Historically marginalized and underrepresented people may have unique concerns and vulnerabilities that need to be considered to ensure their safety and well-being. By providing appropriate safeguards, such as trained facilitators, clear consent practices, and trauma-informed approaches, we can help minimize potential harm and maximize the therapeutic potential of the psychedelic experience.

3. Representation and Diversity

Historically marginalized and underrepresented communities bring diverse perspectives, insights, and experiences to *every* table. By actively promoting inclusivity and diversity in psychedelic and ancestral medicine spaces, we enhance the richness and effectiveness of the therapeutic process. Representation matters, and when people from underrepresented groups feel seen, heard, and valued, it fosters a sense of belonging and facilitates multi-generational healing.

4. Empowerment and Agency

Ancestral Medicine experiences can be empowering and transformative. These experiences can be particularly impactful in restoring agency and self-empowerment. By prioritizing the protection and empowerment of historically marginalized and underrepresented individuals, we can create opportunities for personal growth, self-discovery, and healing that can extend beyond the experience and flow into families, society, and the world.

5. Ethical Considerations

In the field of psychedelic-assisted therapy and research, ethical considerations are paramount. It is important to uphold the following principles: autonomy, respect, beneficence, and justice. We uphold these ethical principles by ensuring that everyone is protected and included, allowing us to work toward a more equitable and just society.

By addressing historical imbalances, creating safe environments, promoting diversity, and empowering individuals, we can harness the full potential of psychedelics for healing and personal growth.

EXAMPLES OF HARM IN MEDICINE SPACES

There is an enormous amount of vulnerability when in an altered state. I aim to offer advice on how (we can collectively) keep each other safe. The types of harm that I am *most* concerned about include:

- **Rape/sexual assault**
- **Emotional abuse/verbal abuse/bullying**
- **Physical violence/ aggression/assault**
- **Non-consensual communication or touch**
- **Flirting, invasive, or inappropriate comments/conversations**
- **"Consensual sex" between medicine facilitator/participant (inside and outside of medicine spaces)**
- **Altered-state sex in medicine spaces without previous consent during the non-altered-state**
- **Non-disclosure and non-consent regarding medicine dosing**
- **Intimidation/threats/harassment/fear tactics**
- **Stalking**
- **Grooming**
- **Coercion**
- **Identity erasure**
- **Identity slurs**
- **Leadership/community alignment w/ predators**
- **Community silence/rejection/alienation**
- **Denial of harm/trauma**
- **All forms of abuse/harm/misconduct not listed above**

Although we cannot fully guarantee safety or prevent all forms of abuse, here are a few suggestions to keep in mind *before* a medicine experience:

- Go into each group medicine experience with solidarity and support for one another.
- Be aware of the power imbalance that exists in medicine spaces.
- Discuss consent regarding touch, space, body autonomy, nudity, relationship, and communication outside of the ceremony.
- Go into healing practices and ceremonies with people who you know and trust.
- Engage in healing practices and ceremonies with experienced people.
- Work with people and organizations who have a zero-tolerance policy against discrimination, harassment, and race/gender/sexual identity-based harm.
- Trust your intuition.
- Ask questions, even the uncomfortable or difficult ones.
- Give yourself permission to cancel medicine experiences, internships, or training at the first, second, or third(+) sign of discomfort — trust your inner knowing.
- Ask if you can bring an escort you trust — especially if you will be in a solo or 1:1 experience. If the answer is *no*, ask for justification and consider whether this is acceptable or safe.
- Know that you have rights regardless of the medicine space or legality. You do not have to remain silent about abuse.
- Know that if the alleged abuser is trained or certified by a professional organization, you can report the abuse to that licensed organization and law enforcement.

If harm happens, here are a few actions that you can take:

- If you see something or experience something, *say* something. Remember that if something happens to one person, it happens to us all. Reporting saves lives.
- Hold a community meeting or circle to discuss the event and explore a plan of action.
- Consider meeting with a Restorative Justice Facilitator for accountability, justice, and non-punitive actions.
- Within a safe community, address what led to the harm and how to decrease the chances of a recurrence in the future.

QUESTIONS TO ASK THE MEDICINE FACILITATOR

- Will you be sending an informed consent document?
- Who is facilitating the medicine?
- Who else will be present?
- How many helpers or trip sitters (i.e., people who offer emotional, spiritual, or physical support while in an altered state) will be present during my medicine experience?
- How many people will be in a sober/non-altered state?
- How many people will be in an altered state while the medicine is being administered?
- How do you plan to ensure safety?
- What groups will be represented (e.g., socioeconomic, age, ability, culture, religion, race, gender, sexuality)?
- Where/When/Who trained you?
- Have you had any ruptures with others, and if so, how did you handle it?
- If a rupture happens between us, how will you address it?
- Have you ever been accused of sexual abuse, misconduct, or any ethical violations?
- Have you had any charges, convictions, or arrests?
- Has your professional license or certification ever been revoked?
- Have you ever been sued?
- Regarding healing touch/therapeutic touch — what does this mean to you?
- How do you address boundaries and consent before and during an altered-state experience?
    - Now is the time to discuss your needs as they relate to boundaries with space, touch, language, preference of gender/sexuality of facilitator or sitter, etc.
- Have you ever been accused of being racist, sexist, homophobic, or transphobic?
- What is your relationship with the LGBTQIA+ and Transgender community?
- How do you address the needs of the Neurodiverse and disability community?
- What is your relationship with people who hold underrepresented identities?
- What is your relationship with the medicine?
- What does your inner work (i.e., mental, emotional, and spiritual) include?

- What are the risks or considerations when taking psychedelic and ancestral medicine?
- What happens during a scary or overwhelming journey, and how will I be cared for during the experience?
- In case of a medical or mental health emergency, how will you address this?

PRE-INTEGRATION CONVERSATION TOPICS

- What was your first introduction to psychedelic and ancestral medicine?
- What are your needs, and how are you taking care of the following:

    - Medical
    - Mental/Emotional
    - Physical
    - Spiritual
    - Social
    - Intellectual
    - Financial
    - Occupational
    - Environmental

- What do your parts need to feel safe in your medicine experience?
- Are there any accommodations that you will need?
- How do you handle strong emotions in your daily life?
- Do your parts have specific needs for lighting, space, sounds, touch, or smell?
- Do your parts have specific emotional or somatic triggers that should be explored before the medicine experience?
- What is your preferred communication style (e.g., verbal, in writing, movement, or other methods)?
- Are there specific ways that you would like to receive information or communication during an altered-state experience (e.g., slower speech, visual aids, etc.)?
- Do your parts prefer being in a group setting or solitude during the altered-state experience?
- Are there specific types of social dynamics that make your parts feel supported or stressed?
- Have you had any previous medicine experiences that were painful or traumatic?
- What would you need if the experience becomes unsafe, scary, overwhelming, or uncomfortable?
- How do your parts like to integrate emotionally or spiritually (e.g., peer support group, one-on-one, journaling, therapy, or coaching)?
- Are there any spiritual or cultural practices that you would like to incorporate?

- How do you experience marginalization or underrepresentation in your day-to-day life?
- Is there anything that needs to be explored regarding identity, power, and privilege?
- Are there particular ways you feel your intersecting identities (i.e., race, gender, sexuality, religion, neurodiversity, and more) might affect your medicine experience?
- Who is on your emergency contacts list?
- Are your parts open to unexpected outcomes, both positive and challenging?

"We have five different elements: earth, water, mineral, fire, and nature. The element earth is responsible for our groundedness, our sense of identity, and our ability to nurture and to support one another. Water is peace, focus, wisdom, and reconciliation. Mineral helps us to remember our purpose and gives us the means to communicate and to make sense out of what others are saying. Fire is about dreaming, keeping our connection to the self and ancestors and keeping our visions alive. Nature helps us to be our true self, to go through major changes and life-threatening situations. It brings magic and laughter."

~SOBONFU SOMÉ

SELF-QUALITIES

In the Internal Family Systems model, Dr. Richard Swartz lists the following as self-energy qualities:

- **Courage**
- **Compassion**
- **Clarity**
- **Confidence**
- **Curiosity**
- **Creativity**
- **Connectedness**
- **Calmness**

After training in Internal Family Systems Level One training, I immediately started to consider other qualities of self that originate in the African American community and the African Diaspora. My heart took me on a path of exploring Kwanzaa, a holiday developed by cultural activist Maulana Karenga and others in the 1960s. In the book, "Practicing Kwanzaa Year Round," Gwynelle Dismukes informs readers that the holiday is structured around seven principles aimed at Black self-awareness and empowerment. The seven principles are as follows:

Umoja **(unity):** to be forgiving and compassionate with one another. To strive for (and maintain) unity in family, community, race, and nation.

Kujichagulia **(self-determination):** to build self-discipline to attain power and realize one's full potential.

Ujima **(collective work and responsibility):** to build and keep our community together, to make our brothers' and sisters' problems *our* problems, and to solve them together.

Ujamaa **(cooperative economics):** to build and manage our own stores, shops, and other businesses and profit from them together.

Nia **(purpose):** to understand one's unique role in the community and how it contributes to the collective purpose.

Kuumba **(creativity):** to always do as much as we can (in the way we can) to leave our community more beautiful and beneficial than we inherited it.

Imani **(faith):** to believe with all our heart in our parents, teachers, leaders, our people, and the righteousness and victory of our struggle.

Reading the principles of Kwanzaa gave me great pride and clarity regarding what (*actually*) heals us individually and collectively — community. The principles reminded me that healing is not a solitary experience. What if the principles of Kwanzaa are qualities of self in the African Diaspora? What are the other qualities of self in the Asian Diaspora, Indigenous, Latine(x) culture, and LGBTQIA+ communities?

As I began brainstorming, I understood that our values, culture, and history intersect and align. I cannot understand parts without honoring my history, *our* collective history. This way of healing our deeply wounded selves began before the creation of IFS, before colonization. One way I want to honor the history of Indigenous communities and the LGBTQIA+ community is by elaborating on other equally important qualities of self. For those of us who belong to the Global Majority, here are the intersectional characteristics that I have noticed:

- **Connection to ancestors**
- **Cultural representation**
- **Rituals of healing**
- **Collective identity**
- **Spirituality**
- **Respect for animals, nature, and community**
- **Storytelling**
- **Balance/mindfulness/meditation**

Our wounded parts reflect the trauma, history, traditions, and resilience of our ancestral lineage. Our healing is a practice of remembering that we are more than trauma—healing is our birthright, and it is in our DNA. People of the Global Majority have known the pain of colonization, oppression, migration, economic instability, and the removal of human rights.

To honor *all* of the communities that I've discussed, here are more qualities of self to consider that honor the Global Majority:

1. **Choice**
2. **Co-creation**
3. **Community**
4. **Cultural Expression**
5. **Comedy/Laughter**
6. **Celebration**
7. **Community Care**
8. **Ceremony**
9. **Consent**
10. **Protection**
11. **Contentment**
12. **Tenderness**
13. **Unity**
14. **Continuity**
15. **Speaking up**
16. **Social Justice**
17. **Anger**

18. **Intuition**
19. **Feminine Erotic Power**
20. **Language**
21. **Emancipation of Oppressive Systems**
22. **Reciprocity**
23. **Nurture**
24. **Queerness**
25. **Passion**
26. **Respect for animals/nature/people**

As you read through this list of inclusive qualities of self, which parts resonate with you? Are there others that come to mind?
_____
_____

"To heal ourselves is to heal the generations that have come before us and to create a ripple effect for the ones that will come after. Our collective healing is imperative in this lifetime. Releasing the ancestral trauma and cultural legacy burdens carried in our minds, bodies, and spirits isn't just some radical and idealistic idea — it's surely our only route to liberation and wholeness."

~NATALIE Y. GUTIÉRREZ,
THE PAIN WE CARRY

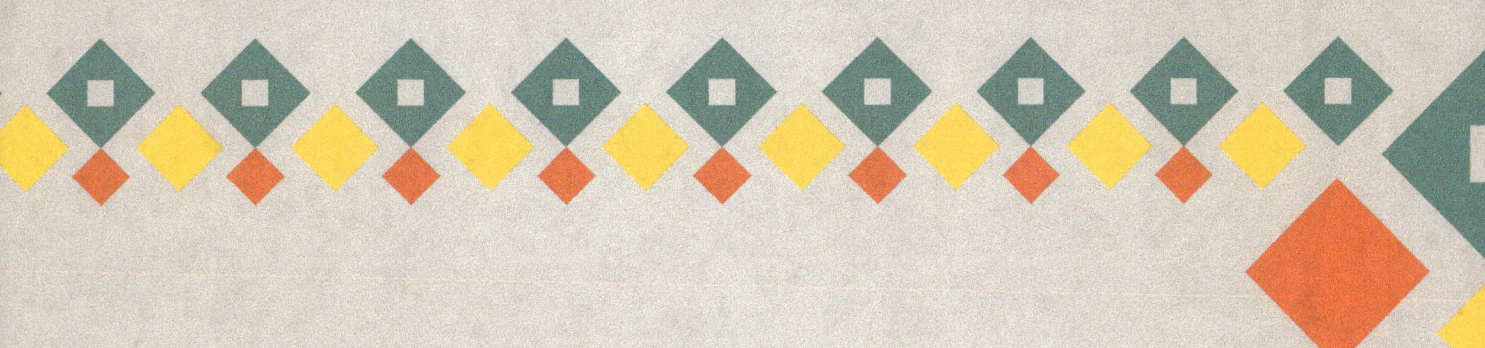

GUIDED JOURNALING WORKSHEET

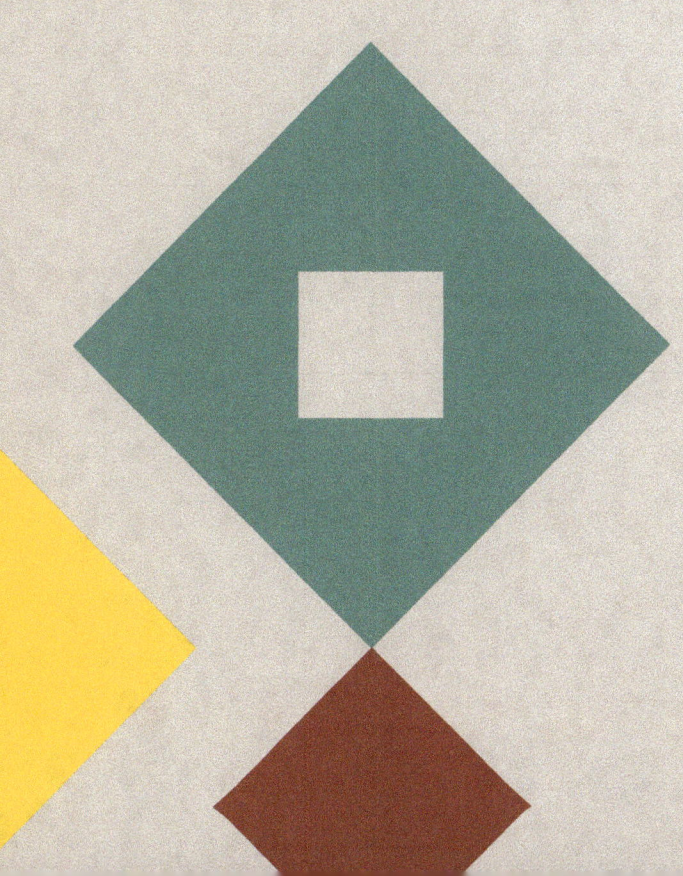

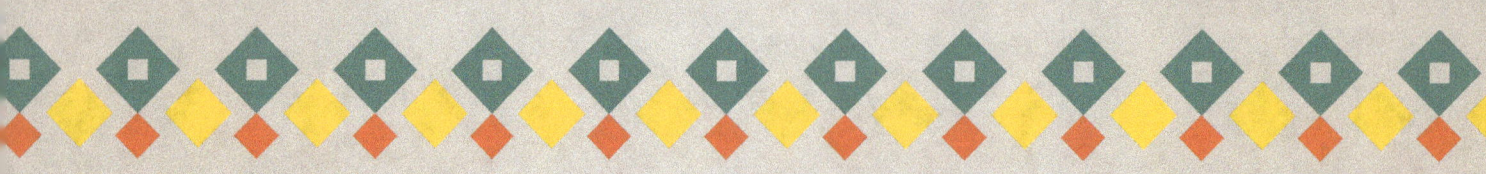

Pre-Integration Date(s): _____   Integration Date(s): _____

Post-Integration Date(s): _____

Start time: _____   End time: _____

Medicine Facilitator: _____   Trip Sitter(s): _____

Therapist/Coach/Spiritual Advisor: _____

Other Supports Present: _____

Group or Individual Experience: _____

Type of Medicine and Dosage: _____

AT THIS MOMENT, I AM FEELING:
_____
_____

AT THIS MOMENT, I AM READY TO RECEIVE:
_____
_____

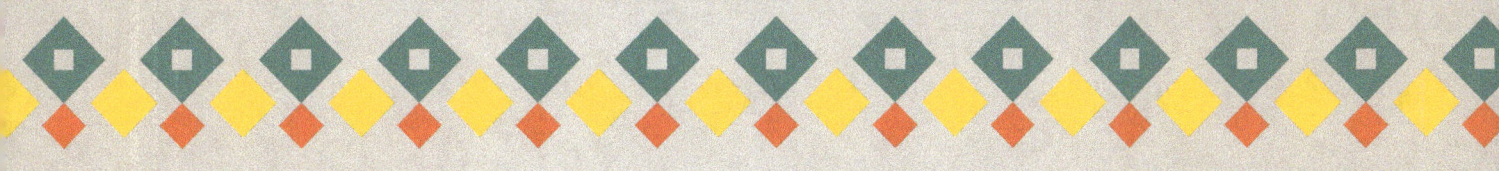

PART'S INTENTIONS:

_____
_____
_____

SELF-ENERGY INTENTIONS:

_____
_____
_____

LIST FEARS OR CONCERNS:

_____
_____
_____

NOTE PEOPLE, PLACES, MEMORIES, THEMES, OR ANYTHING ELSE THAT YOU WOULD LIKE TO REMEMBER ABOUT YOUR MEDICINE EXPERIENCE:

_____
_____
_____
_____
_____

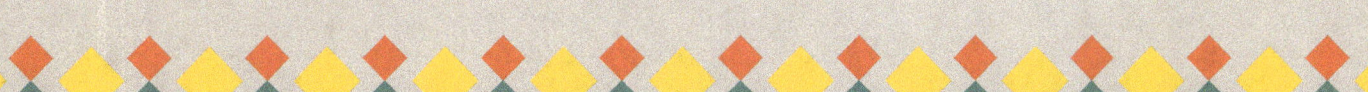

SCENES MY PARTS REVEALED DURING THE MEDICINE EXPERIENCE:
_____
_____

THOUGHTS DURING THE EXPERIENCE:
_____
_____
_____

WHAT CHANGES DID I NOTICE WITHIN MY BODY
AFTER THE MEDICINE ADMINISTRATION?
_____
_____

LIST ANY OTHER SENSATIONS PRESENT:
_____
_____

PARTS THAT SHOWED UP DURING THE MEDICINE EXPERIENCE:
_____   _____
_____   _____

SELF-ENERGY QUALITIES PRESENT DURING THE EXPERIENCE:
_____
_____
_____

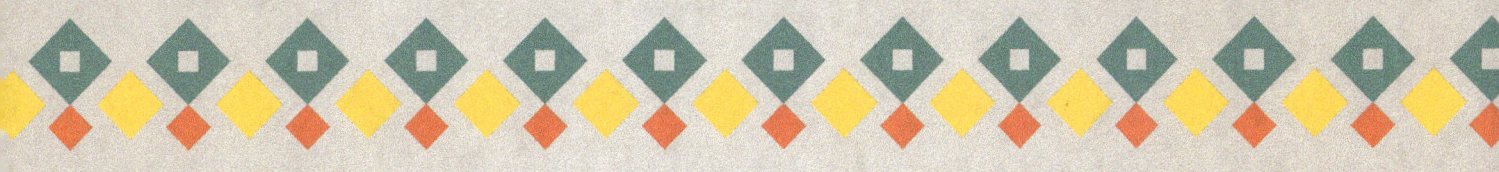

BURDENS REVEALED (E.G., PERSONAL, CULTURAL, OR ANCESTRAL, GLOBAL):
_____
_____
_____

ANCESTORS PRESENT:
_____   _____
_____   _____

SPIRIT GUIDES:
_____   _____
_____   _____

EARTHLY ELEMENTS THAT WERE A PART OF THE EXPERIENCE:

☐ Water   ☐ Metal   ☐ Force
☐ Mineral   ☐ Wood   ☐ Shadow
☐ Fire   ☐ Plants   ☐ Light
☐ Air   ☐ Time   ☐ Sun/Moon

WHAT FELT MOST CHALLENGING?
_____
_____

GUIDED JOURNALING WORKSHEET

IF YOU EXPERIENCED AN OVERWHELMING OR SCARY JOURNEY — WHAT PARTS WERE ACTIVATED?

_____
_____
_____

WHAT FELT MOST REWARDING?

_____
_____

KEY INSIGHTS OR CURIOSITIES:

_____
_____
_____

BURDENS REVEALED:

_____
_____
_____

WERE ANY PARTS *UNBURDENED*?

_____
_____

DID THE MESSAGES THAT YOUR PARTS SHARED MAKE SENSE TO YOU?
_____

WHAT DO YOU PLAN TO INTEGRATE?
_____
_____
_____

WHAT GIFTS, PARTS, OR LESSONS ARE YOU TAKING WITH YOU?
_____
_____

THE TARGET PART FOR MY POST-INTEGRATION SESSIONS WILL BE:
_____
_____

GUIDED JOURNALING WORKSHEET

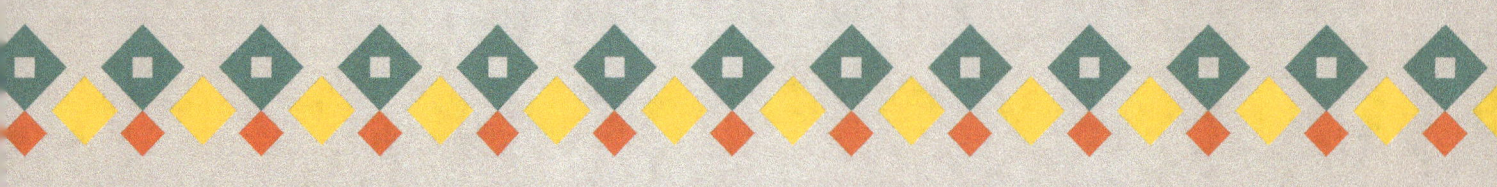

JOURNALING PAGE

_____
_____
_____
_____
_____
_____
_____
_____
_____
_____
_____
_____
_____
_____
_____
_____
_____
_____

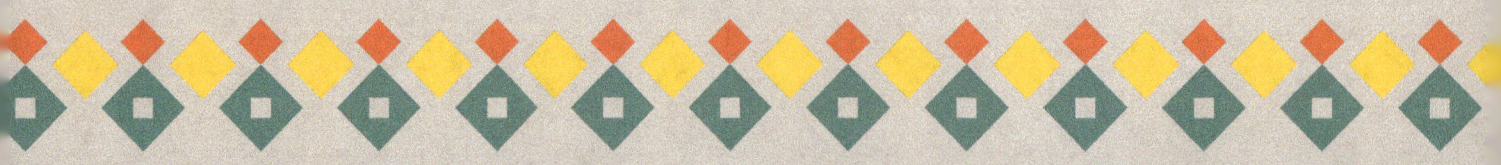

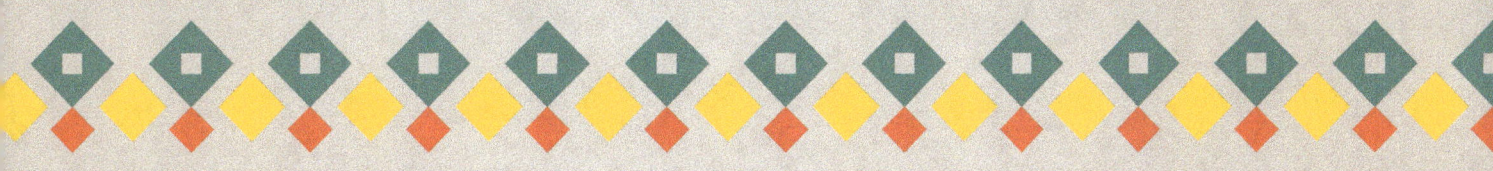

PARTS MAPPING

Close your eyes and imagine that you are landing inside of yourself, where you can clearly feel the presence of your parts.

What do you notice?

Is there a part that feels most present or alive? Using the prompts below, draw and journal your responses below on the following pages.

1. **Part's Name**
2. **Part's Purpose/Role**
3. **Part's Emotion/Feeling/Thoughts**
4. **Somatic Location of Part**
5. **Part's fears, anxieties, or concerns**
6. **Part's Characteristics (i.e., color, shape, size, sound, age, energy)**
7. **What do you need each part to know about you?**
8. **Is the part a protector (i.e., manager or firefighter) or an exile?**
9. **What else does the part need you to know about it?**

PARTS MAPPING SPACE

PARTS MAPPING SPACE

"Are you sure, sweetheart, that you want to be well?… Just so's you're sure, sweetheart, and ready to be healed, cause wholeness is no trifling matter. A lot of weight when you're well."

~TONI CADE BAMBARA, THE SALT EATERS

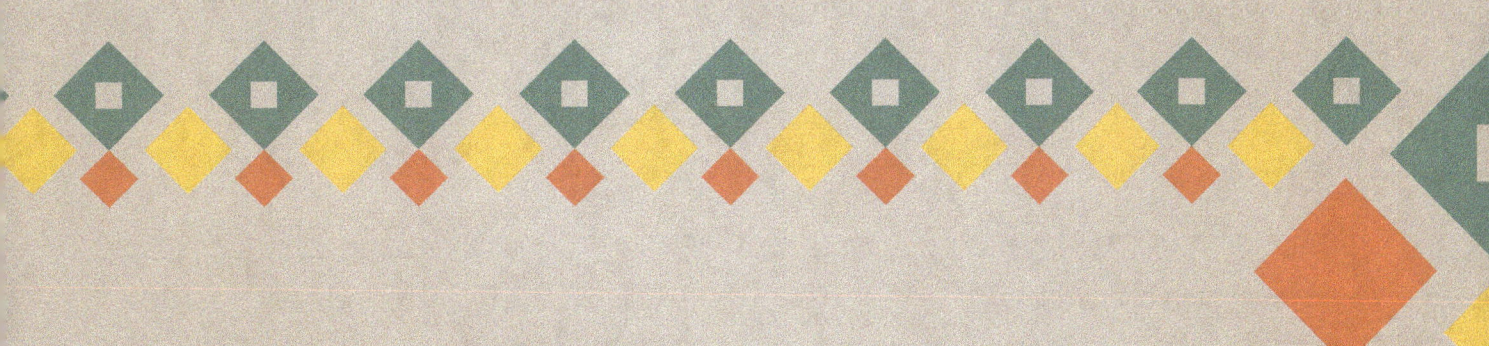

GUIDED JOURNALING WORKSHEET

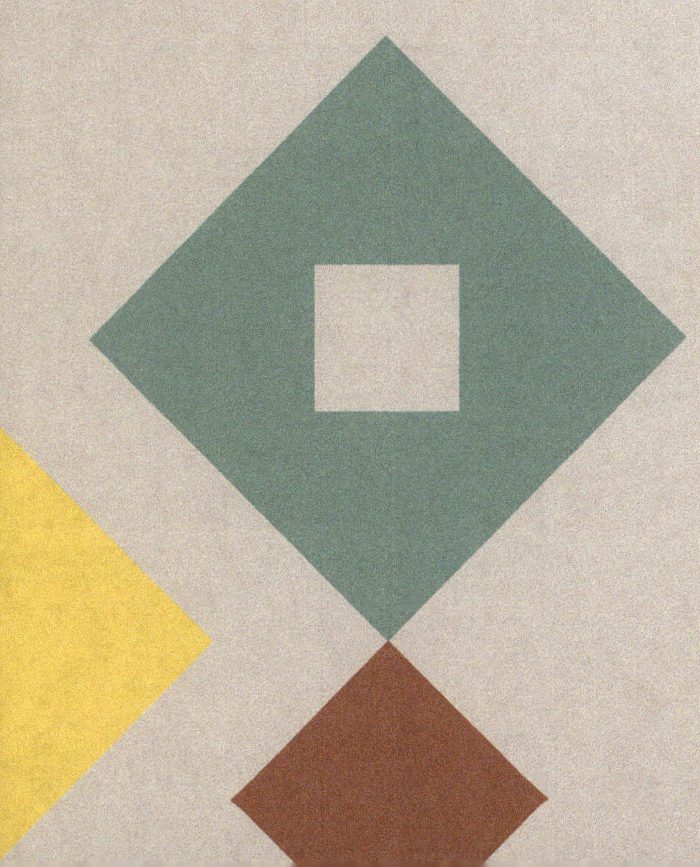

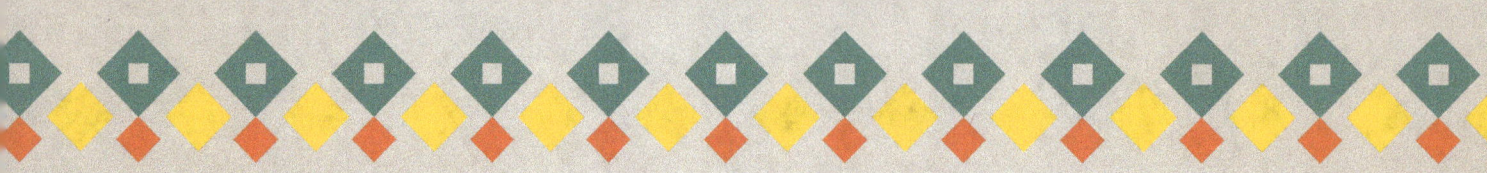

Pre-Integration Date(s): _____   Integration Date(s): _____

Post-Integration Date(s): _____

Start time: _____   End time: _____

Medicine Facilitator: _____   Trip Sitter(s): _____

Therapist/Coach/Spiritual Advisor: _____

Other Supports Present: _____

Group or Individual Experience: _____

Type of Medicine and Dosage: _____

AT THIS MOMENT, I AM FEELING:
_____
_____

AT THIS MOMENT, I AM READY TO RECEIVE:
_____
_____

LIBERATION

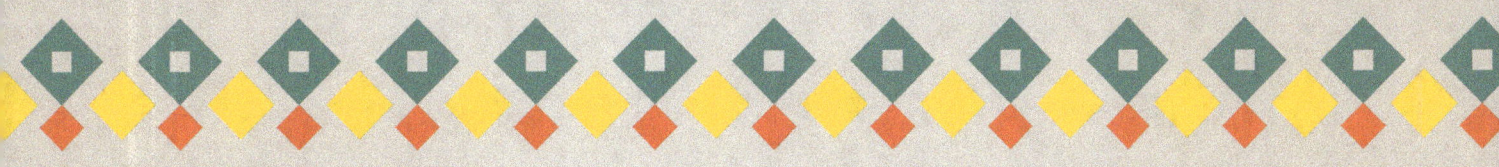

PART'S INTENTIONS:
_____
_____
_____

SELF-ENERGY INTENTIONS:
_____
_____
_____
_____

LIST FEARS OR CONCERNS:
_____
_____
_____
_____

NOTE PEOPLE, PLACES, MEMORIES, THEMES, OR ANYTHING ELSE THAT YOU WOULD LIKE TO REMEMBER ABOUT YOUR MEDICINE EXPERIENCE:
_____
_____
_____
_____
_____
_____

GUIDED JOURNALING WORKSHEET

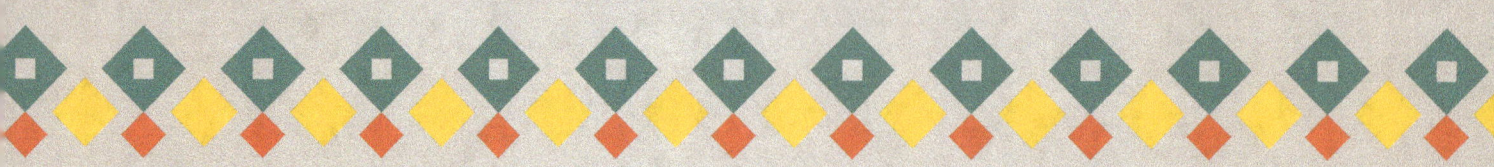

SCENES MY PARTS REVEALED DURING THE MEDICINE EXPERIENCE:
_____
_____

THOUGHTS DURING THE EXPERIENCE:
_____
_____
_____

WHAT CHANGES DID I NOTICE WITHIN MY BODY
AFTER THE MEDICINE ADMINISTRATION?
_____
_____

LIST ANY OTHER SENSATIONS PRESENT:
_____
_____

PARTS THAT SHOWED UP DURING THE MEDICINE EXPERIENCE:
_____   _____
_____   _____

SELF-ENERGY QUALITIES PRESENT DURING THE EXPERIENCE:
_____
_____
_____

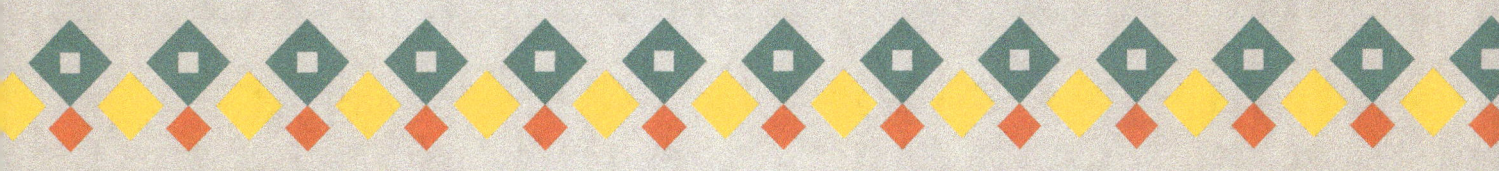

BURDENS REVEALED (E.G., PERSONAL, CULTURAL, OR ANCESTRAL, GLOBAL):
_____
_____
_____

ANCESTORS PRESENT:
_____   _____
_____   _____

SPIRIT GUIDES:
_____   _____
_____   _____

EARTHLY ELEMENTS THAT WERE A PART OF THE EXPERIENCE:

- ☐ Water
- ☐ Mineral
- ☐ Fire
- ☐ Air
- ☐ Metal
- ☐ Wood
- ☐ Plants
- ☐ Time
- ☐ Force
- ☐ Shadow
- ☐ Light
- ☐ Sun/Moon

WHAT FELT MOST CHALLENGING?
_____
_____

GUIDED JOURNALING WORKSHEET

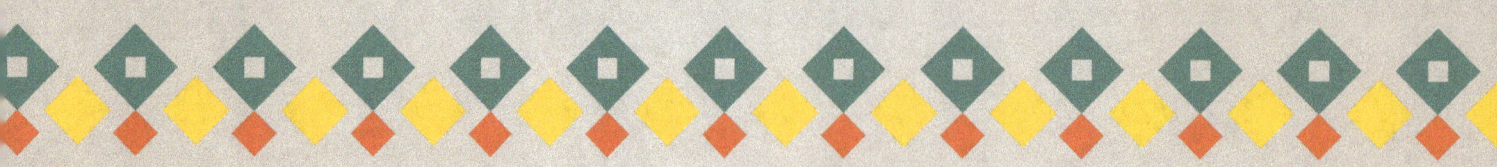

IF YOU EXPERIENCED AN OVERWHELMING OR SCARY JOURNEY — WHAT PARTS WERE ACTIVATED?
_____
_____
_____

WHAT FELT MOST REWARDING?
_____
_____

KEY INSIGHTS OR CURIOSITIES:
_____
_____
_____

BURDENS REVEALED:
_____
_____
_____

WERE ANY PARTS *UNBURDENED*?
_____
_____

DID THE MESSAGES THAT YOUR PARTS SHARED MAKE SENSE TO YOU?

WHAT DO YOU PLAN TO INTEGRATE?

WHAT GIFTS, PARTS, OR LESSONS ARE YOU TAKING WITH YOU?

THE TARGET PART FOR MY POST-INTEGRATION SESSIONS WILL BE:

JOURNALING PAGE

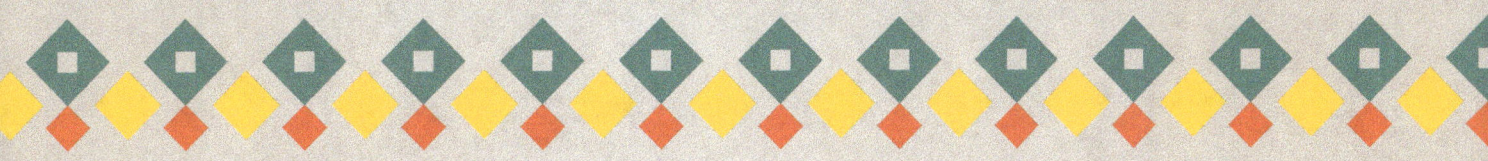

PARTS MAPPING

Close your eyes and imagine that you are landing inside of yourself, where you can clearly feel the presence of your parts.

What do you notice?

Is there a part that feels most present or alive? Using the prompts below, draw and journal your responses below on the following pages.

1. **Part's Name**
2. **Part's Purpose/Role**
3. **Part's Emotion/Feeling/Thoughts**
4. **Somatic Location of Part**
5. **Part's fears, anxieties, or concerns**
6. **Part's Characteristics (i.e., color, shape, size, sound, age, energy)**
7. **What do you need each part to know about you?**
8. **Is the part a protector (i.e., manager or firefighter) or an exile?**
9. **What else does the part need you to know about it?**

PARTS MAPPING SPACE

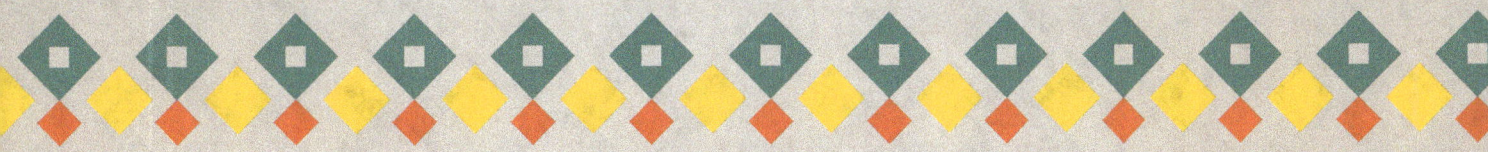

PARTS MAPPING SPACE

"I pray I've done my work so, that when I've gone from here, in all the turmoil through the wreckage and rumble, when someone finds themselves digging through the ruins, they'll find me. Somewhere in that wreckage, they'll find something they can use, that I left behind. And if I've done that, then I've accomplished something in life."

~JAMES BALDWIN

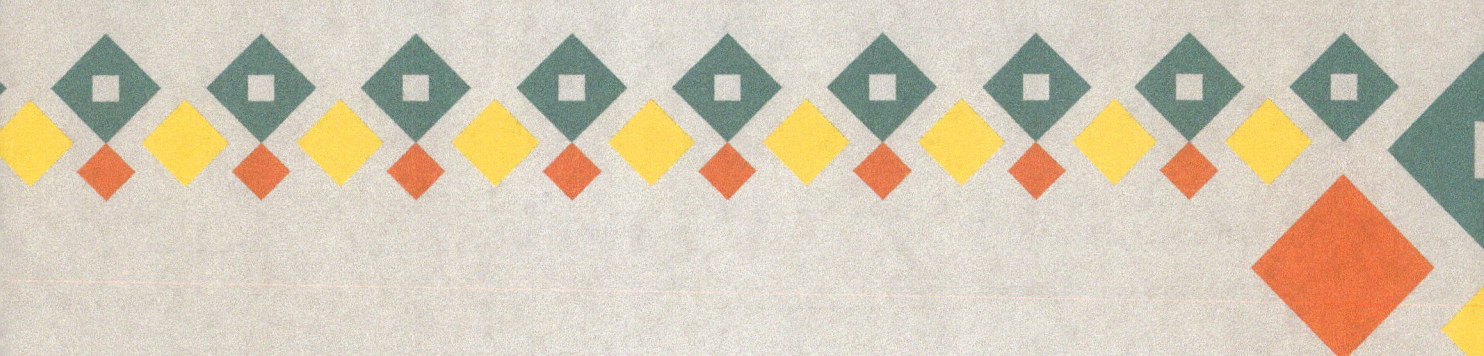

GUIDED JOURNALING WORKSHEET

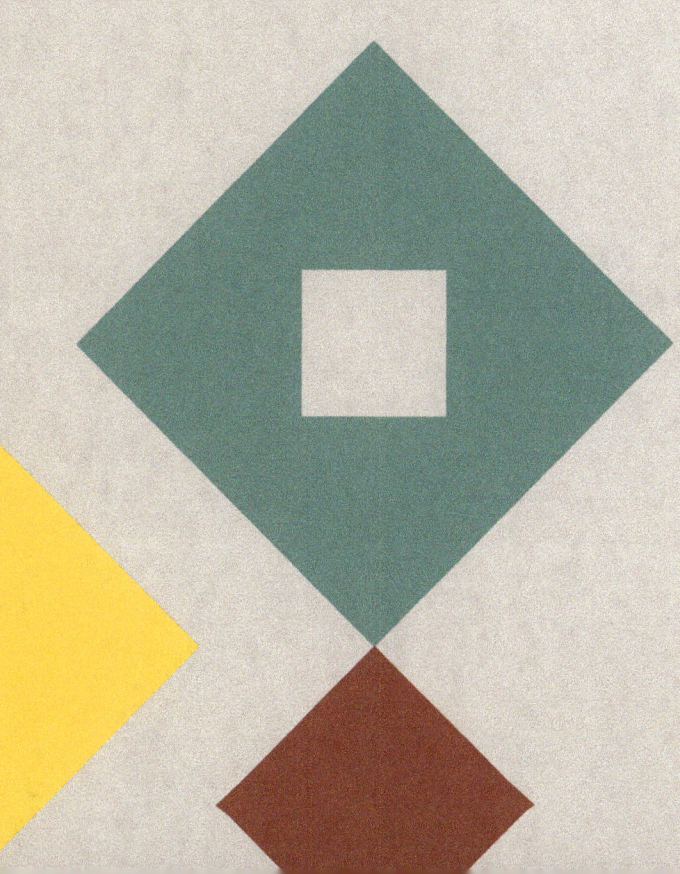

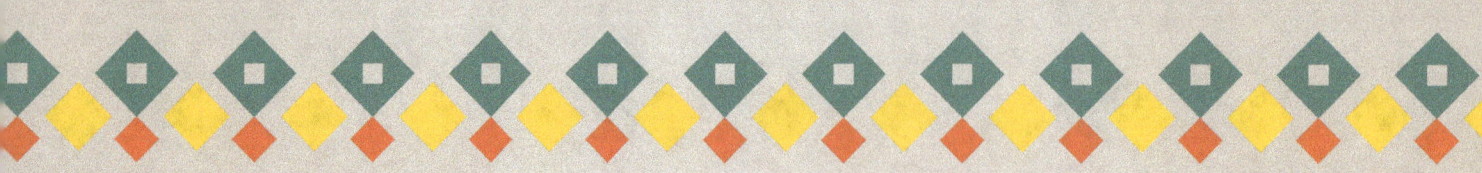

Pre-Integration Date(s): _____   Integration Date(s): _____

Post-Integration Date(s): _____

Start time: _____   End time: _____

Medicine Facilitator: _____   Trip Sitter(s): _____

Therapist/Coach/Spiritual Advisor: _____

Other Supports Present: _____

Group or Individual Experience: _____

Type of Medicine and Dosage: _____

AT THIS MOMENT, I AM FEELING:
_____
_____

AT THIS MOMENT, I AM READY TO RECEIVE:
_____
_____

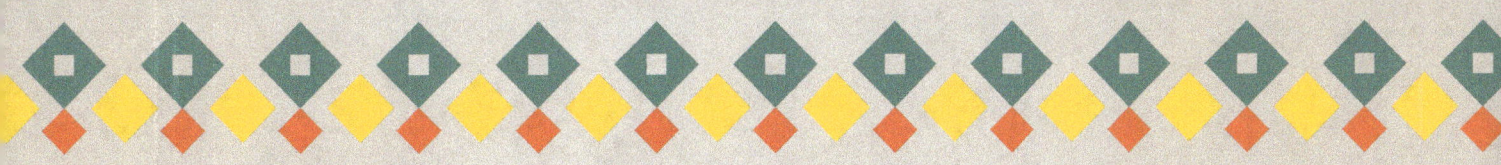

PART'S INTENTIONS:
_____
_____
_____

SELF-ENERGY INTENTIONS:
_____
_____
_____

LIST FEARS OR CONCERNS:
_____
_____
_____

NOTE PEOPLE, PLACES, MEMORIES, THEMES, OR ANYTHING ELSE THAT YOU WOULD LIKE TO REMEMBER ABOUT YOUR MEDICINE EXPERIENCE:
_____
_____
_____
_____
_____

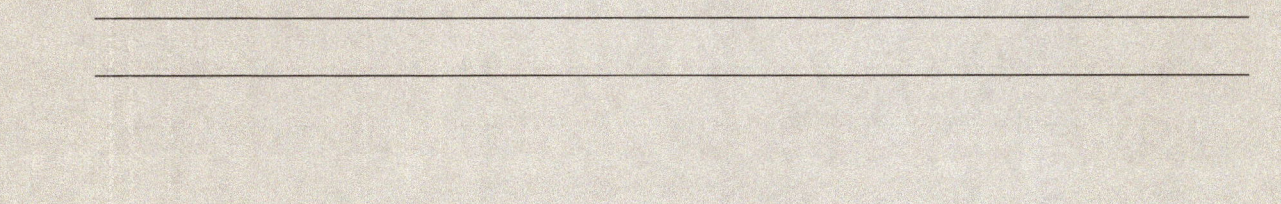

SCENES MY PARTS REVEALED DURING THE MEDICINE EXPERIENCE:
_____
_____

THOUGHTS DURING THE EXPERIENCE:
_____
_____
_____

WHAT CHANGES DID I NOTICE WITHIN MY BODY
AFTER THE MEDICINE ADMINISTRATION?
_____
_____

LIST ANY OTHER SENSATIONS PRESENT:
_____
_____

PARTS THAT SHOWED UP DURING THE MEDICINE EXPERIENCE:
_____   _____
_____   _____

SELF-ENERGY QUALITIES PRESENT DURING THE EXPERIENCE:
_____
_____
_____

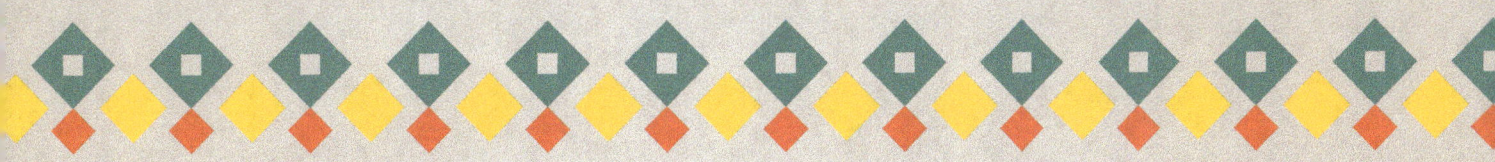

BURDENS REVEALED (E.G., PERSONAL, CULTURAL, OR ANCESTRAL, GLOBAL):

_____
_____
_____

ANCESTORS PRESENT:

_____ _____
_____ _____

SPIRIT GUIDES:

_____ _____
_____ _____

EARTHLY ELEMENTS THAT WERE A PART OF THE EXPERIENCE:

- ☐ Water
- ☐ Mineral
- ☐ Fire
- ☐ Air
- ☐ Metal
- ☐ Wood
- ☐ Plants
- ☐ Time
- ☐ Force
- ☐ Shadow
- ☐ Light
- ☐ Sun/Moon

WHAT FELT MOST CHALLENGING?

_____
_____

IF YOU EXPERIENCED AN OVERWHELMING OR SCARY JOURNEY — WHAT PARTS WERE ACTIVATED?

_____
_____
_____

WHAT FELT MOST REWARDING?

_____
_____

KEY INSIGHTS OR CURIOSITIES:

_____
_____
_____

BURDENS REVEALED:

_____
_____
_____

WERE ANY PARTS *UNBURDENED?*

_____
_____

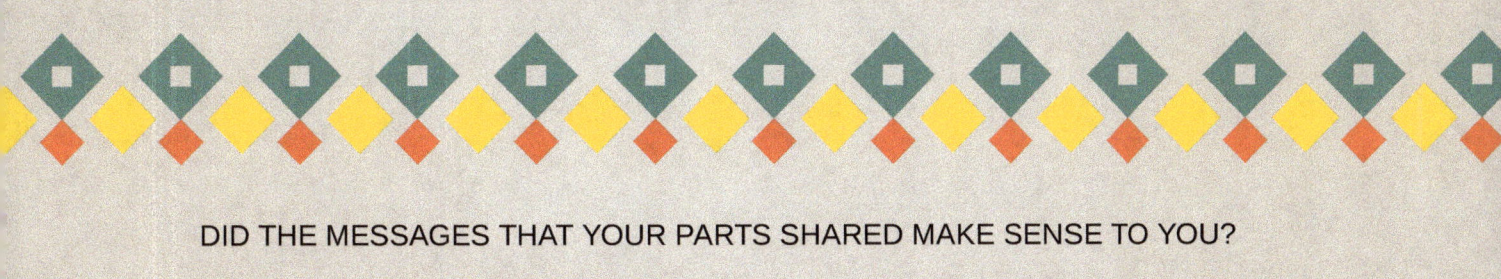

DID THE MESSAGES THAT YOUR PARTS SHARED MAKE SENSE TO YOU?
_____

WHAT DO YOU PLAN TO INTEGRATE?
_____
_____
_____

WHAT GIFTS, PARTS, OR LESSONS ARE YOU TAKING WITH YOU?
_____
_____
_____

THE TARGET PART FOR MY POST-INTEGRATION SESSIONS WILL BE:
_____
_____

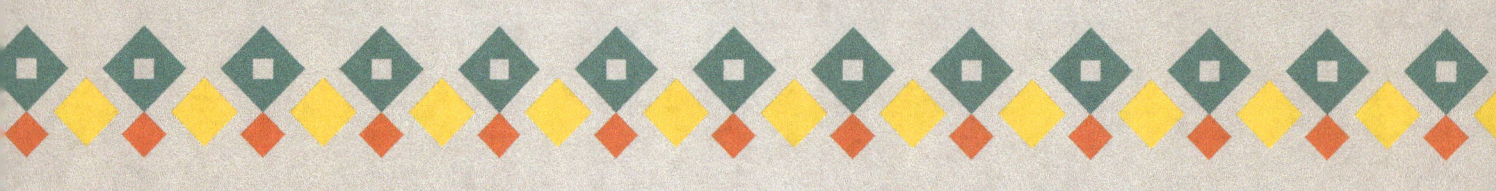

JOURNALING PAGE

_____
_____
_____
_____
_____
_____
_____
_____
_____
_____
_____
_____
_____
_____
_____
_____
_____
_____

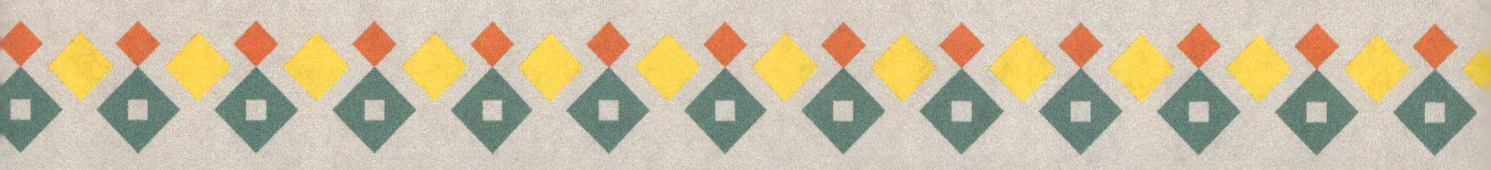

PARTS MAPPING

Close your eyes and imagine that you are landing inside of yourself, where you can clearly feel the presence of your parts.

What do you notice?

Is there a part that feels most present or alive? Using the prompts below, draw and journal your responses below on the following pages.

1. **Part's Name**
2. **Part's Purpose/Role**
3. **Part's Emotion/Feeling/Thoughts**
4. **Somatic Location of Part**
5. **Part's fears, anxieties, or concerns**
6. **Part's Characteristics (i.e., color, shape, size, sound, age, energy)**
7. **What do you need each part to know about you?**
8. **Is the part a protector (i.e., manager or firefighter) or an exile?**
9. **What else does the part need you to know about it?**

PARTS MAPPING SPACE

PARTS MAPPING SPACE

"*Courage is the most important of all the virtues because, without courage, you can't practice any other virtue consistently.*"

~MAYA ANGELOU

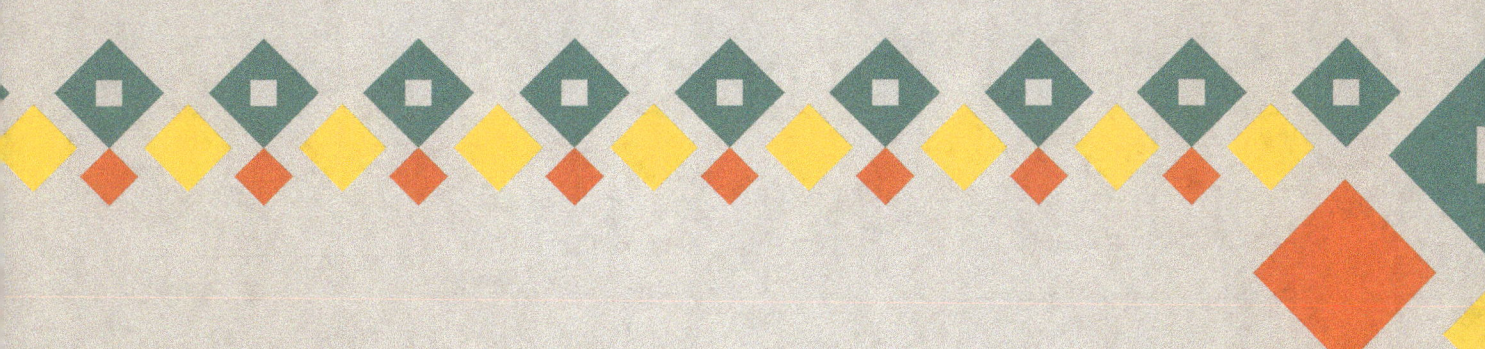

GUIDED JOURNALING WORKSHEET

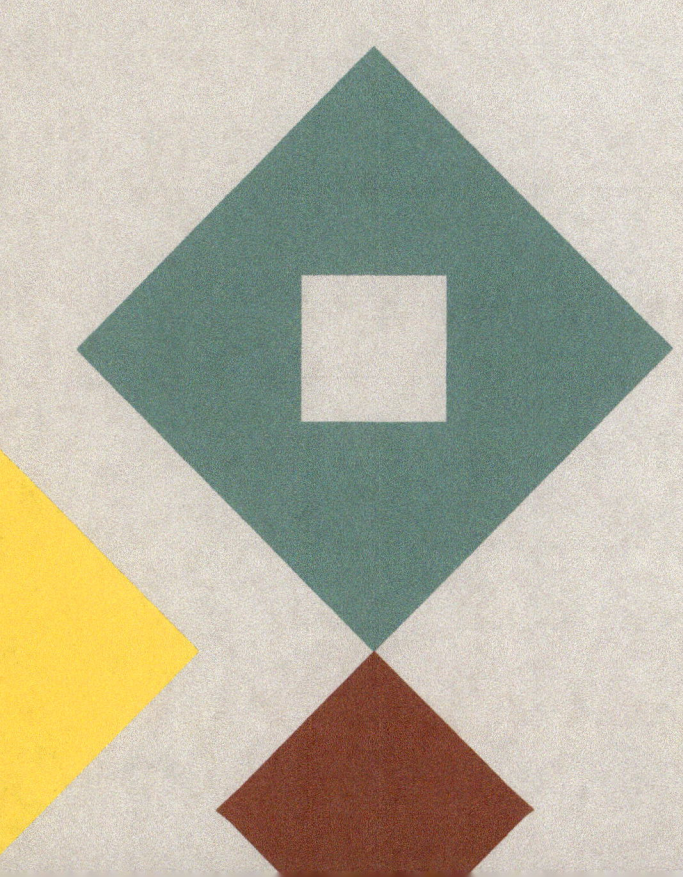

Pre-Integration Date(s): _____   Integration Date(s): _____

Post-Integration Date(s): _____

Start time: _____   End time: _____

Medicine Facilitator: _____   Trip Sitter(s): _____

Therapist/Coach/Spiritual Advisor: _____

Other Supports Present: _____

Group or Individual Experience: _____

Type of Medicine and Dosage: _____

```
┌─────────────────────────────────────────────────────────────┐
│              AT THIS MOMENT, I AM FEELING:                  │
│   _____  │
│   _____  │
└─────────────────────────────────────────────────────────────┘
```

```
┌─────────────────────────────────────────────────────────────┐
│           AT THIS MOMENT, I AM READY TO RECEIVE:            │
│   _____  │
│   _____  │
└─────────────────────────────────────────────────────────────┘
```

PART'S INTENTIONS:
_____
_____
_____

SELF-ENERGY INTENTIONS:
_____
_____
_____
_____

LIST FEARS OR CONCERNS:
_____
_____
_____
_____

NOTE PEOPLE, PLACES, MEMORIES, THEMES, OR ANYTHING ELSE THAT YOU WOULD LIKE TO REMEMBER ABOUT YOUR MEDICINE EXPERIENCE:
_____
_____
_____
_____
_____
_____

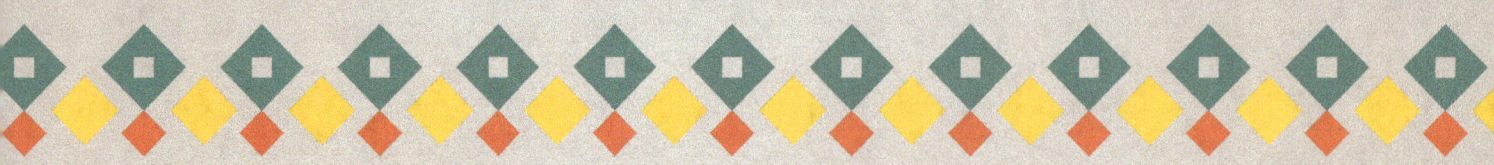

SCENES MY PARTS REVEALED DURING THE MEDICINE EXPERIENCE:
_____
_____

THOUGHTS DURING THE EXPERIENCE:
_____
_____
_____

WHAT CHANGES DID I NOTICE WITHIN MY BODY
AFTER THE MEDICINE ADMINISTRATION?
_____
_____

LIST ANY OTHER SENSATIONS PRESENT:
_____
_____

PARTS THAT SHOWED UP DURING THE MEDICINE EXPERIENCE:
_____   _____
_____   _____

SELF-ENERGY QUALITIES PRESENT DURING THE EXPERIENCE:
_____
_____
_____

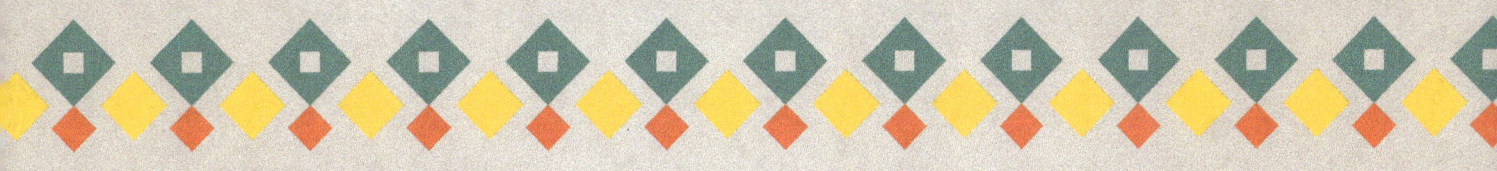

BURDENS REVEALED (E.G., PERSONAL, CULTURAL, OR ANCESTRAL, GLOBAL):
_____
_____
_____

ANCESTORS PRESENT:
_____ _____
_____ _____

SPIRIT GUIDES:
_____ _____
_____ _____

EARTHLY ELEMENTS THAT WERE A PART OF THE EXPERIENCE:

- ☐ Water
- ☐ Mineral
- ☐ Fire
- ☐ Air
- ☐ Metal
- ☐ Wood
- ☐ Plants
- ☐ Time
- ☐ Force
- ☐ Shadow
- ☐ Light
- ☐ Sun/Moon

WHAT FELT MOST CHALLENGING?
_____
_____

IF YOU EXPERIENCED AN OVERWHELMING OR SCARY JOURNEY — WHAT PARTS WERE ACTIVATED?

_____
_____
_____

WHAT FELT MOST REWARDING?

_____
_____

KEY INSIGHTS OR CURIOSITIES:

_____
_____
_____

BURDENS REVEALED:

_____
_____
_____

WERE ANY PARTS *UNBURDENED*?

_____
_____

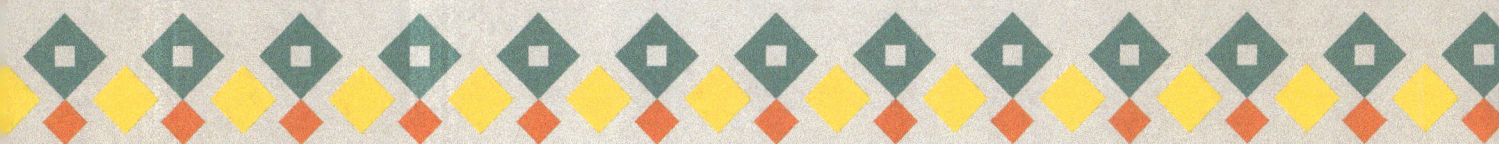

DID THE MESSAGES THAT YOUR PARTS SHARED MAKE SENSE TO YOU?
_____

WHAT DO YOU PLAN TO INTEGRATE?
_____
_____
_____

WHAT GIFTS, PARTS, OR LESSONS ARE YOU TAKING WITH YOU?
_____
_____

THE TARGET PART FOR MY POST-INTEGRATION SESSIONS WILL BE:
_____
_____

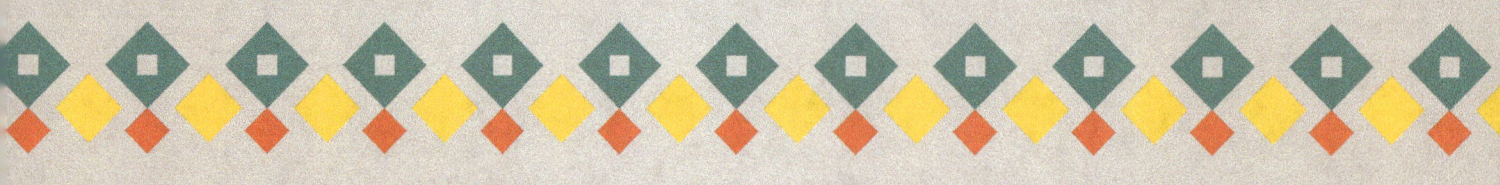

JOURNALING PAGE

_____
_____
_____
_____
_____
_____
_____
_____
_____
_____
_____
_____
_____
_____
_____
_____
_____
_____
_____

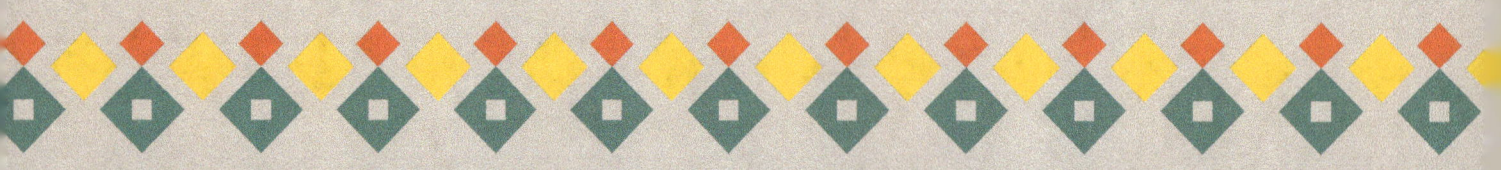

PARTS MAPPING

Close your eyes and imagine that you are landing inside of yourself, where you can clearly feel the presence of your parts.

What do you notice?

Is there a part that feels most present or alive? Using the prompts below, draw and journal your responses below on the following pages.

1. **Part's Name**
2. **Part's Purpose/Role**
3. **Part's Emotion/Feeling/Thoughts**
4. **Somatic Location of Part**
5. **Part's fears, anxieties, or concerns**
6. **Part's Characteristics (i.e., color, shape, size, sound, age, energy)**
7. **What do you need each part to know about you?**
8. **Is the part a protector (i.e., manager or firefighter) or an exile?**
9. **What else does the part need you to know about it?**

PARTS MAPPING SPACE

PARTS MAPPING SPACE

"I think that little by little I'll be able to solve my problems and survive."

~FRIDA KAHLO

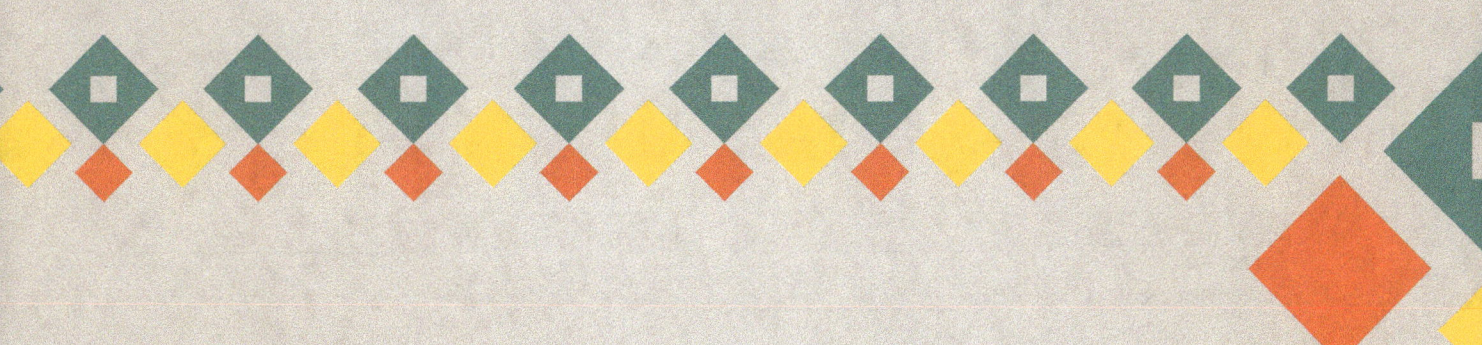

GUIDED JOURNALING WORKSHEET

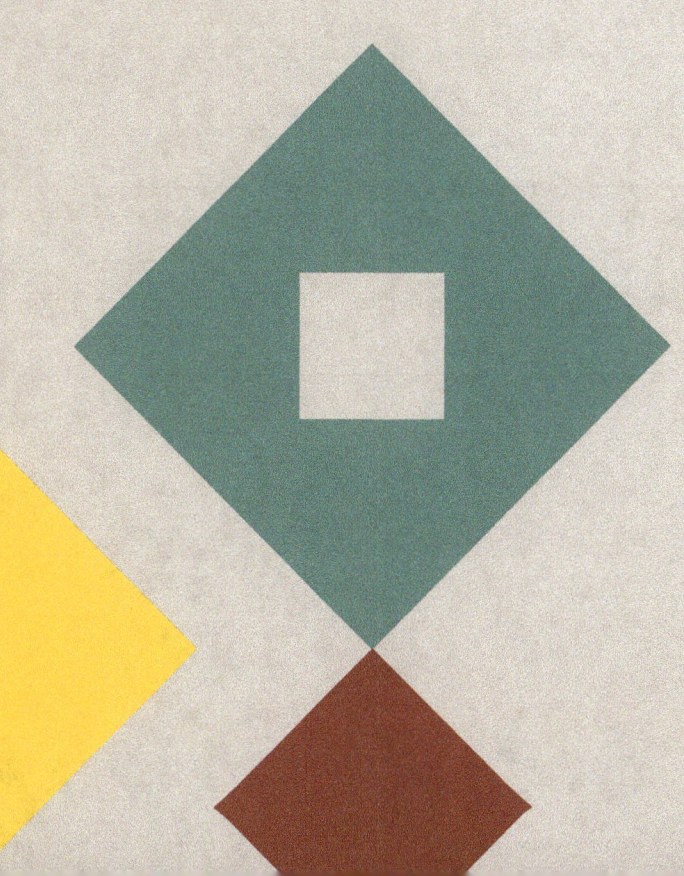

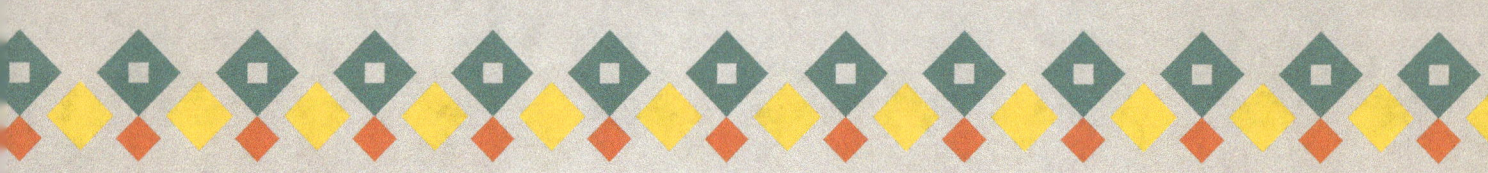

Pre-Integration Date(s): _____ Integration Date(s): _____

Post-Integration Date(s): _____

Start time: _____ End time: _____

Medicine Facilitator: _____ Trip Sitter(s): _____

Therapist/Coach/Spiritual Advisor: _____

Other Supports Present: _____

Group or Individual Experience: _____

Type of Medicine and Dosage: _____

AT THIS MOMENT, I AM FEELING:
_____
_____

AT THIS MOMENT, I AM READY TO RECEIVE:
_____
_____

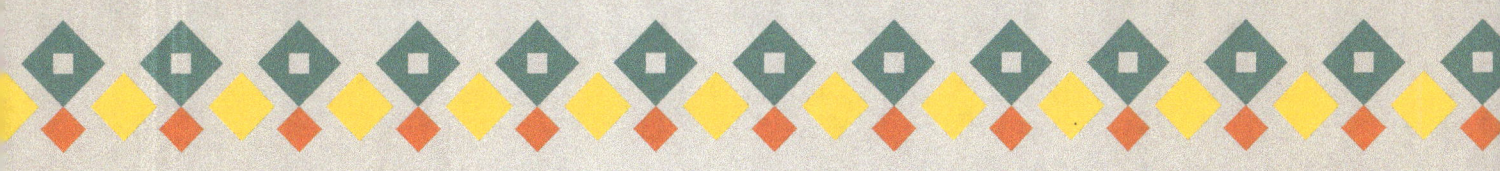

PART'S INTENTIONS:
_____
_____
_____

SELF-ENERGY INTENTIONS:
_____
_____
_____

LIST FEARS OR CONCERNS:
_____
_____
_____
_____

NOTE PEOPLE, PLACES, MEMORIES, THEMES, OR ANYTHING ELSE THAT YOU WOULD LIKE TO REMEMBER ABOUT YOUR MEDICINE EXPERIENCE:
_____
_____
_____
_____
_____
_____

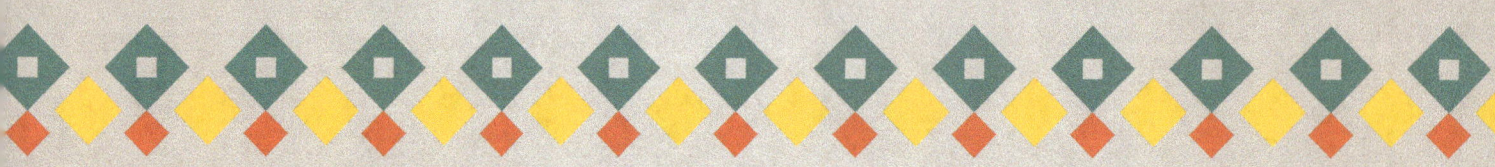

SCENES MY PARTS REVEALED DURING THE MEDICINE EXPERIENCE:
_____
_____

THOUGHTS DURING THE EXPERIENCE:
_____
_____
_____

WHAT CHANGES DID I NOTICE WITHIN MY BODY
AFTER THE MEDICINE ADMINISTRATION?
_____
_____

LIST ANY OTHER SENSATIONS PRESENT:
_____
_____

PARTS THAT SHOWED UP DURING THE MEDICINE EXPERIENCE:
_____   _____
_____   _____

SELF-ENERGY QUALITIES PRESENT DURING THE EXPERIENCE:
_____
_____
_____

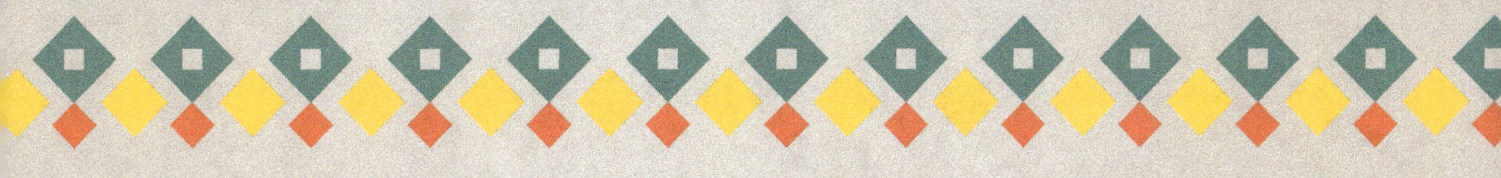

BURDENS REVEALED (E.G., PERSONAL, CULTURAL, OR ANCESTRAL, GLOBAL):
_____
_____
_____

ANCESTORS PRESENT:
_____ _____
_____ _____

SPIRIT GUIDES:
_____ _____
_____ _____

EARTHLY ELEMENTS THAT WERE A PART OF THE EXPERIENCE:

- ☐ Water
- ☐ Mineral
- ☐ Fire
- ☐ Air
- ☐ Metal
- ☐ Wood
- ☐ Plants
- ☐ Time
- ☐ Force
- ☐ Shadow
- ☐ Light
- ☐ Sun/Moon

WHAT FELT MOST CHALLENGING?
_____
_____

GUIDED JOURNALING WORKSHEET

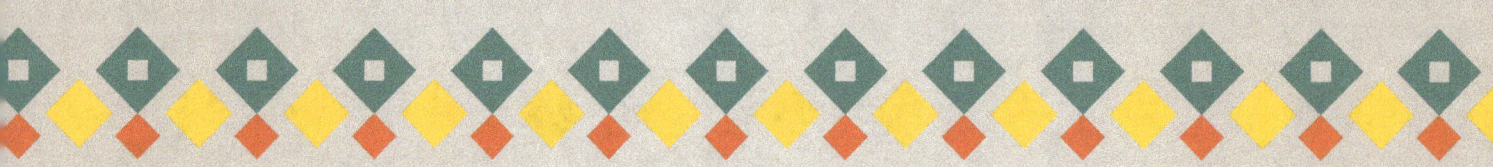

IF YOU EXPERIENCED AN OVERWHELMING OR SCARY JOURNEY — WHAT PARTS WERE ACTIVATED?

_____
_____
_____

WHAT FELT MOST REWARDING?

_____
_____

KEY INSIGHTS OR CURIOSITIES:

_____
_____
_____

BURDENS REVEALED:

_____
_____
_____

WERE ANY PARTS *UNBURDENED?*

_____
_____

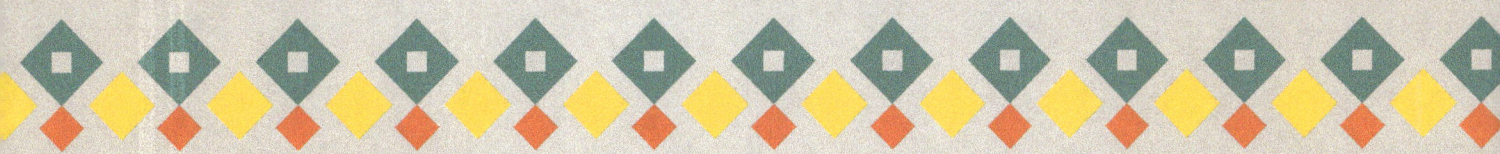

DID THE MESSAGES THAT YOUR PARTS SHARED MAKE SENSE TO YOU?
_____

WHAT DO YOU PLAN TO INTEGRATE?
_____
_____
_____

WHAT GIFTS, PARTS, OR LESSONS ARE YOU TAKING WITH YOU?
_____
_____
_____

THE TARGET PART FOR MY POST-INTEGRATION SESSIONS WILL BE:
_____
_____

GUIDED JOURNALING WORKSHEET

JOURNALING PAGE

PARTS MAPPING

Close your eyes and imagine that you are landing inside of yourself, where you can clearly feel the presence of your parts.

What do you notice?

Is there a part that feels most present or alive? Using the prompts below, draw and journal your responses below on the following pages.

1. **Part's Name**
2. **Part's Purpose/Role**
3. **Part's Emotion/Feeling/Thoughts**
4. **Somatic Location of Part**
5. **Part's fears, anxieties, or concerns**
6. **Part's Characteristics (i.e., color, shape, size, sound, age, energy)**
7. **What do you need each part to know about you?**
8. **Is the part a protector (i.e., manager or firefighter) or an exile?**
9. **What else does the part need you to know about it?**

PARTS MAPPING SPACE

PARTS MAPPING SPACE

"Letting go gives us freedom, and freedom is the only condition for happiness. If in our heart, we still cling to anything — anger, anxiety, or possessions — we cannot be free."

~THICH NHAT HANH

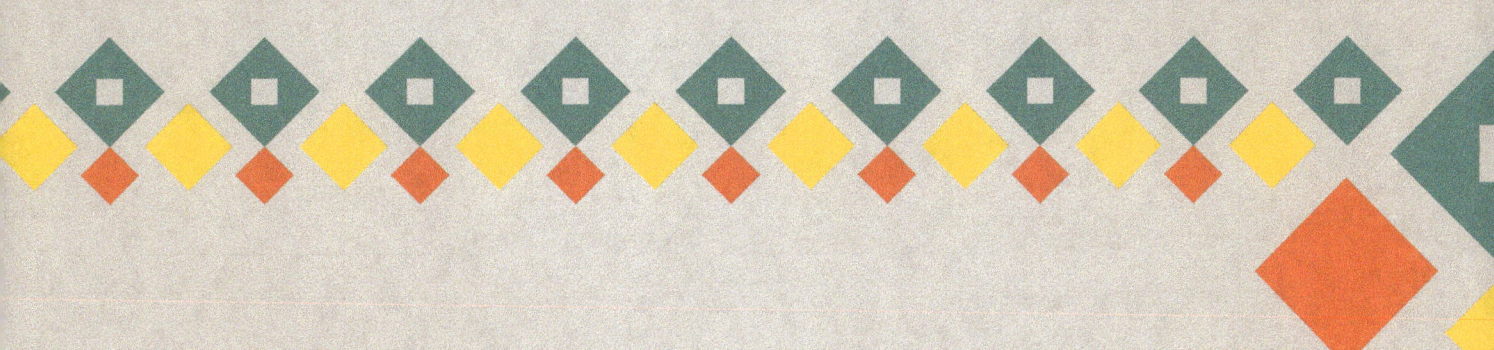

GUIDED JOURNALING WORKSHEET

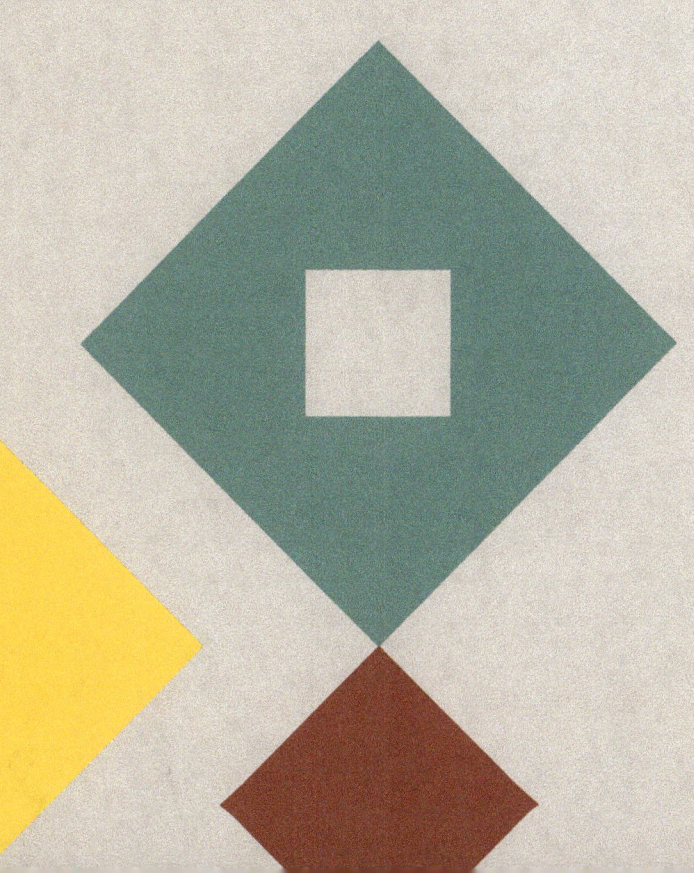

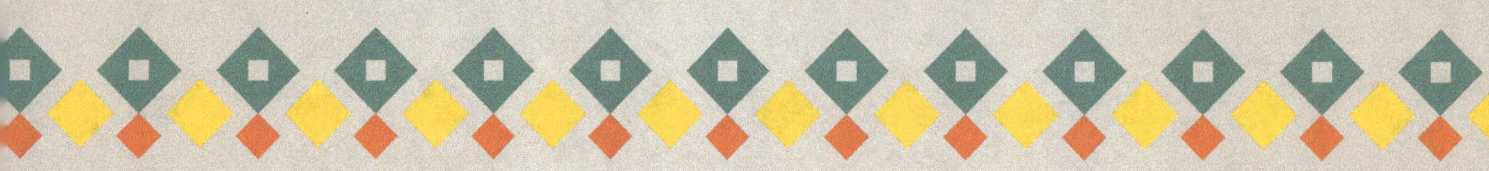

Pre-Integration Date(s): _____ Integration Date(s): _____

Post-Integration Date(s): _____

Start time: _____ End time: _____

Medicine Facilitator: _____ Trip Sitter(s): _____

Therapist/Coach/Spiritual Advisor: _____

Other Supports Present: _____

Group or Individual Experience: _____

Type of Medicine and Dosage: _____

AT THIS MOMENT, I AM FEELING:

_____

_____

AT THIS MOMENT, I AM READY TO RECEIVE:

_____

_____

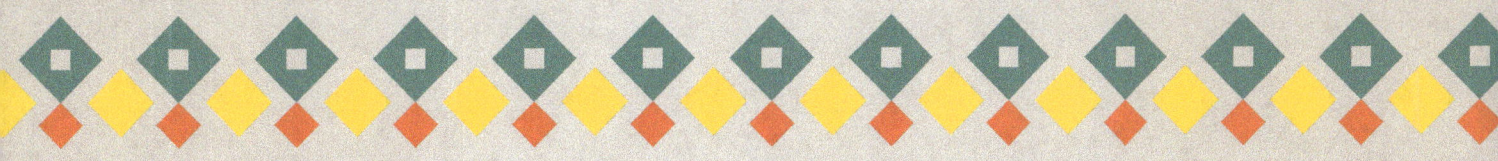

PART'S INTENTIONS:
_____
_____
_____

SELF-ENERGY INTENTIONS:
_____
_____
_____

LIST FEARS OR CONCERNS:
_____
_____
_____

NOTE PEOPLE, PLACES, MEMORIES, THEMES, OR ANYTHING ELSE THAT YOU WOULD LIKE TO REMEMBER ABOUT YOUR MEDICINE EXPERIENCE:
_____
_____
_____
_____
_____
_____

SCENES MY PARTS REVEALED DURING THE MEDICINE EXPERIENCE:
_____
_____

THOUGHTS DURING THE EXPERIENCE:
_____
_____
_____

WHAT CHANGES DID I NOTICE WITHIN MY BODY
AFTER THE MEDICINE ADMINISTRATION?
_____
_____

LIST ANY OTHER SENSATIONS PRESENT:
_____
_____

PARTS THAT SHOWED UP DURING THE MEDICINE EXPERIENCE:
_____   _____
_____   _____

SELF-ENERGY QUALITIES PRESENT DURING THE EXPERIENCE:
_____
_____
_____

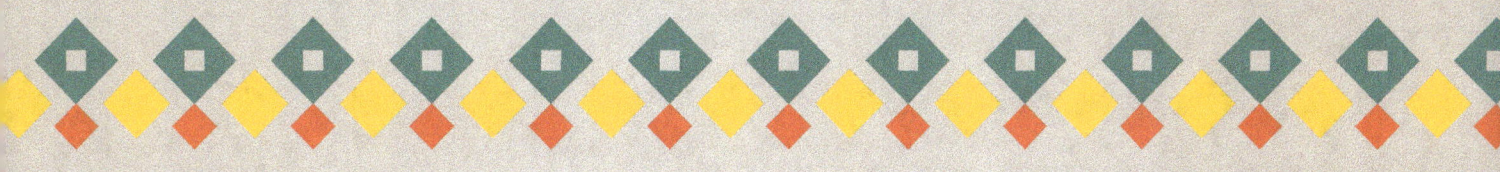

BURDENS REVEALED (E.G., PERSONAL, CULTURAL, OR ANCESTRAL, GLOBAL):
_____
_____
_____

ANCESTORS PRESENT:
_____   _____
_____   _____

SPIRIT GUIDES:
_____   _____
_____   _____

EARTHLY ELEMENTS THAT WERE A PART OF THE EXPERIENCE:

- ☐ Water
- ☐ Mineral
- ☐ Fire
- ☐ Air
- ☐ Metal
- ☐ Wood
- ☐ Plants
- ☐ Time
- ☐ Force
- ☐ Shadow
- ☐ Light
- ☐ Sun/Moon

WHAT FELT MOST CHALLENGING?
_____
_____

GUIDED JOURNALING WORKSHEET

107

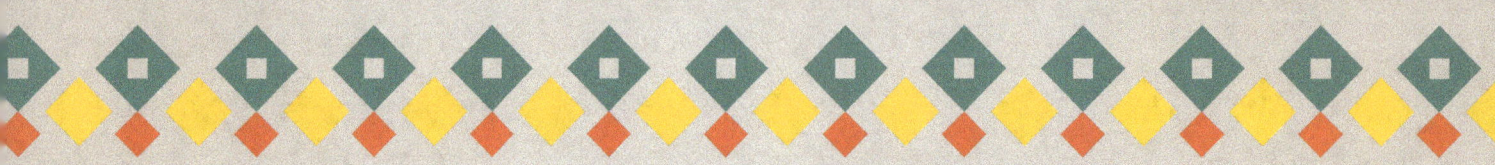

IF YOU EXPERIENCED AN OVERWHELMING OR SCARY JOURNEY — WHAT PARTS WERE ACTIVATED?

_____
_____
_____

WHAT FELT MOST REWARDING?

_____
_____

KEY INSIGHTS OR CURIOSITIES:

_____
_____
_____

BURDENS REVEALED:

_____
_____
_____

WERE ANY PARTS *UNBURDENED?*

_____
_____

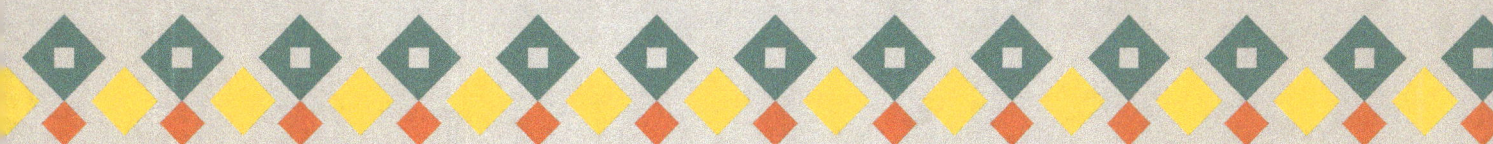

DID THE MESSAGES THAT YOUR PARTS SHARED MAKE SENSE TO YOU?
_____

WHAT DO YOU PLAN TO INTEGRATE?
_____
_____
_____

WHAT GIFTS, PARTS, OR LESSONS ARE YOU TAKING WITH YOU?
_____
_____

THE TARGET PART FOR MY POST-INTEGRATION SESSIONS WILL BE:
_____
_____

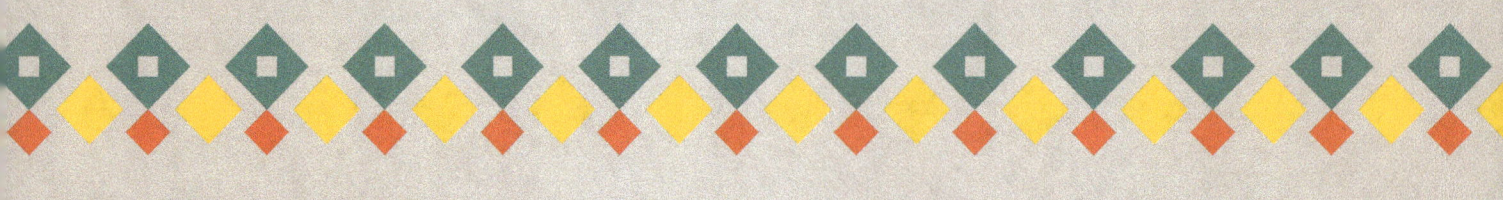

JOURNALING PAGE

_____
_____
_____
_____
_____
_____
_____
_____
_____
_____
_____
_____
_____
_____
_____
_____
_____

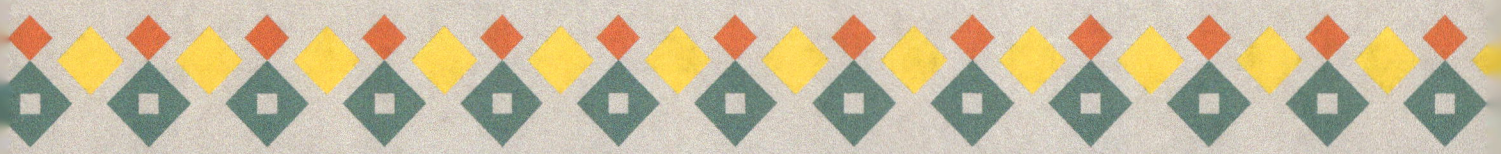

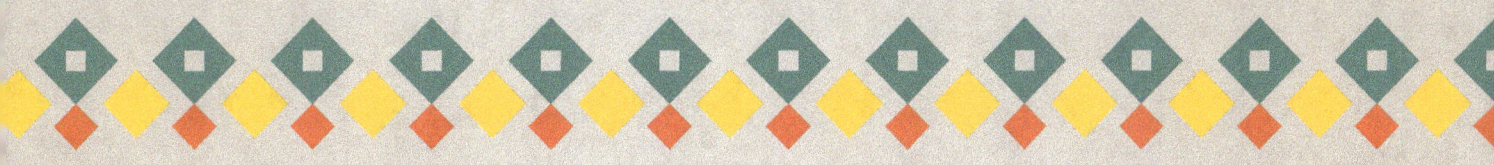

PARTS MAPPING

Close your eyes and imagine that you are landing inside of yourself, where you can clearly feel the presence of your parts.

What do you notice?

Is there a part that feels most present or alive? Using the prompts below, draw and journal your responses below on the following pages.

1. **Part's Name**
2. **Part's Purpose/Role**
3. **Part's Emotion/Feeling/Thoughts**
4. **Somatic Location of Part**
5. **Part's fears, anxieties, or concerns**
6. **Part's Characteristics (i.e., color, shape, size, sound, age, energy)**
7. **What do you need each part to know about you?**
8. **Is the part a protector (i.e., manager or firefighter) or an exile?**
9. **What else does the part need you to know about it?**

PARTS MAPPING SPACE

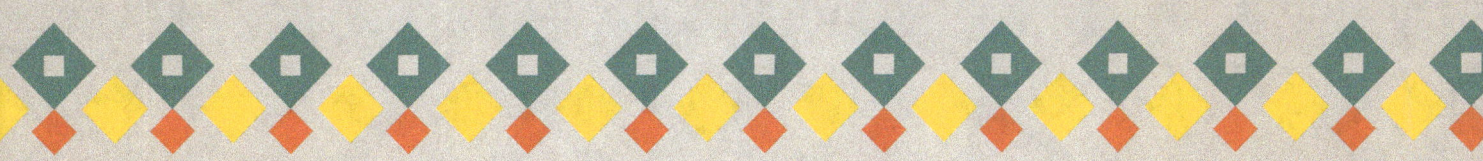

PARTS MAPPING SPACE

"When you dream, you dialogue with aspects of yourself that normally are not with you in the daytime and you discover that you know a great deal more than you thought you did."

~TONI CADE BAMBARA

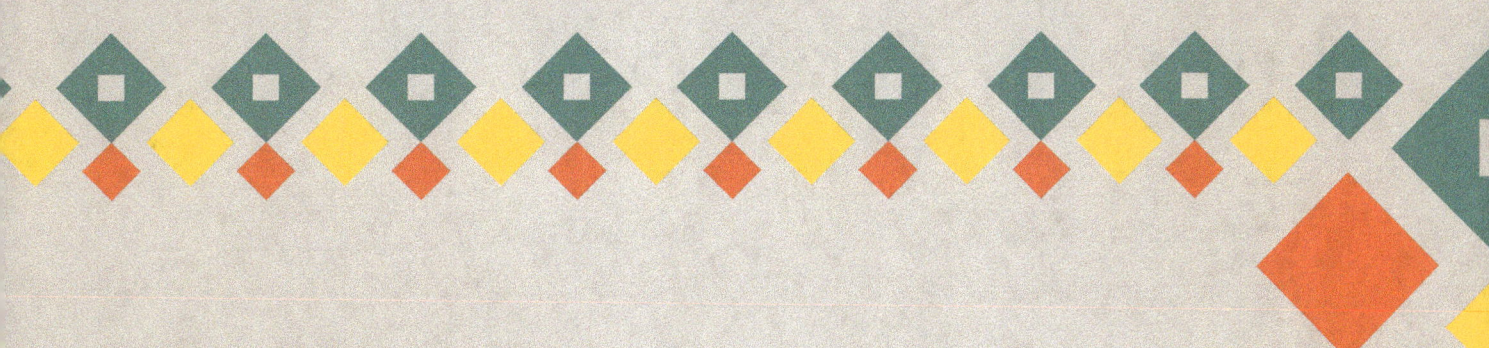

GUIDED JOURNALING WORKSHEET

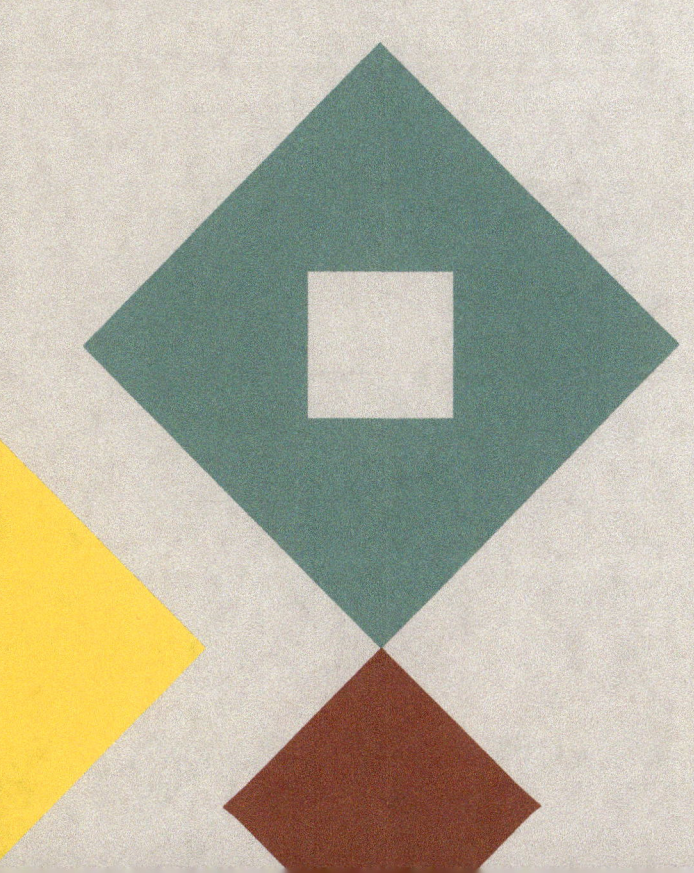

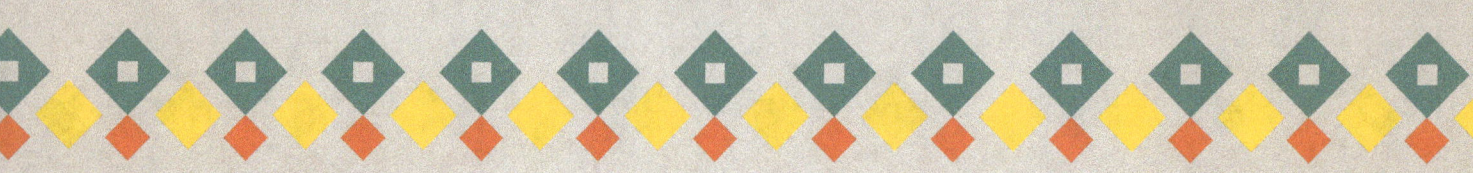

Pre-Integration Date(s): _____ Integration Date(s): _____

Post-Integration Date(s): _____

Start time: _____ End time: _____

Medicine Facilitator: _____ Trip Sitter(s): _____

Therapist/Coach/Spiritual Advisor: _____

Other Supports Present: _____

Group or Individual Experience: _____

Type of Medicine and Dosage: _____

AT THIS MOMENT, I AM FEELING:
_____
_____

AT THIS MOMENT, I AM READY TO RECEIVE:
_____
_____

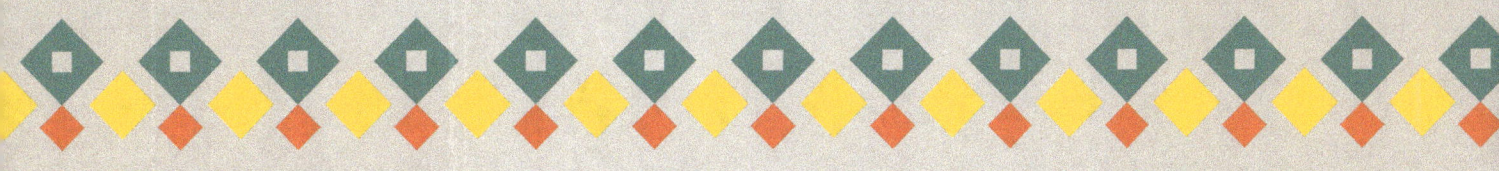

PART'S INTENTIONS:
_____
_____
_____

SELF-ENERGY INTENTIONS:
_____
_____
_____

LIST FEARS OR CONCERNS:
_____
_____
_____

NOTE PEOPLE, PLACES, MEMORIES, THEMES, OR ANYTHING ELSE THAT YOU WOULD LIKE TO REMEMBER ABOUT YOUR MEDICINE EXPERIENCE:
_____
_____
_____
_____
_____

GUIDED JOURNALING WORKSHEET

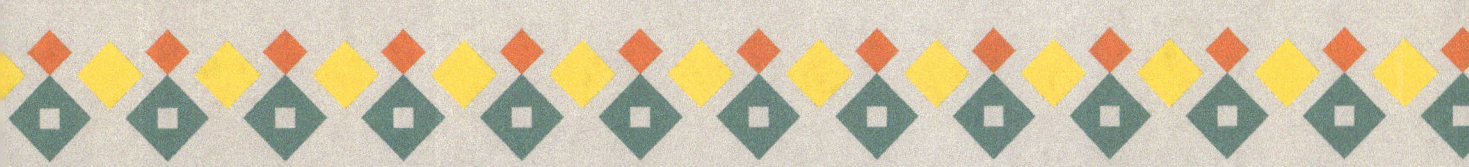

SCENES MY PARTS REVEALED DURING THE MEDICINE EXPERIENCE:
_____
_____

THOUGHTS DURING THE EXPERIENCE:
_____
_____
_____

WHAT CHANGES DID I NOTICE WITHIN MY BODY
AFTER THE MEDICINE ADMINISTRATION?
_____
_____

LIST ANY OTHER SENSATIONS PRESENT:
_____
_____

PARTS THAT SHOWED UP DURING THE MEDICINE EXPERIENCE:
_____   _____
_____   _____

SELF-ENERGY QUALITIES PRESENT DURING THE EXPERIENCE:
_____
_____
_____

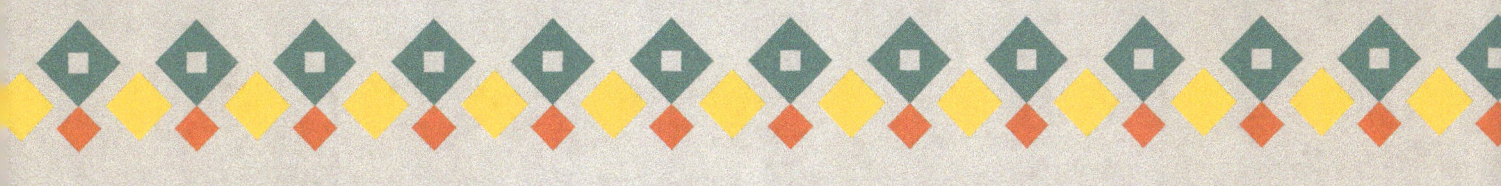

BURDENS REVEALED (E.G., PERSONAL, CULTURAL, OR ANCESTRAL, GLOBAL):
_____
_____
_____

ANCESTORS PRESENT:
_____   _____
_____   _____

SPIRIT GUIDES:
_____   _____
_____   _____

EARTHLY ELEMENTS THAT WERE A PART OF THE EXPERIENCE:

- ☐ Water   ☐ Metal   ☐ Force
- ☐ Mineral   ☐ Wood   ☐ Shadow
- ☐ Fire   ☐ Plants   ☐ Light
- ☐ Air   ☐ Time   ☐ Sun/Moon

WHAT FELT MOST CHALLENGING?
_____
_____

IF YOU EXPERIENCED AN OVERWHELMING OR SCARY JOURNEY — WHAT PARTS WERE ACTIVATED?

_____
_____
_____

WHAT FELT MOST REWARDING?

_____
_____

KEY INSIGHTS OR CURIOSITIES:

_____
_____
_____

BURDENS REVEALED:

_____
_____
_____

WERE ANY PARTS *UNBURDENED?*

_____
_____

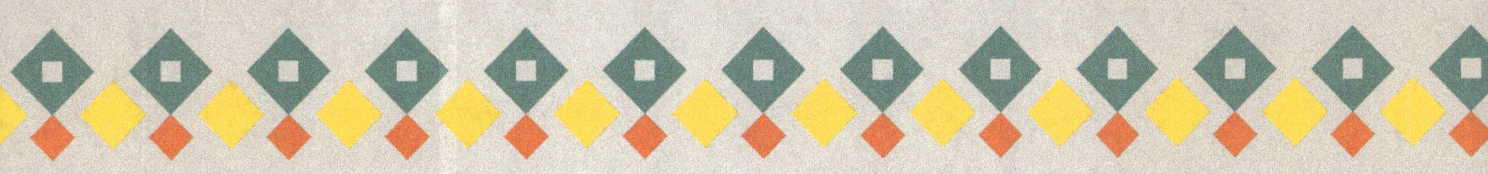

DID THE MESSAGES THAT YOUR PARTS SHARED MAKE SENSE TO YOU?
_____

WHAT DO YOU PLAN TO INTEGRATE?
_____
_____
_____

WHAT GIFTS, PARTS, OR LESSONS ARE YOU TAKING WITH YOU?
_____
_____
_____

THE TARGET PART FOR MY POST-INTEGRATION SESSIONS WILL BE:
_____
_____

GUIDED JOURNALING WORKSHEET

JOURNALING PAGE

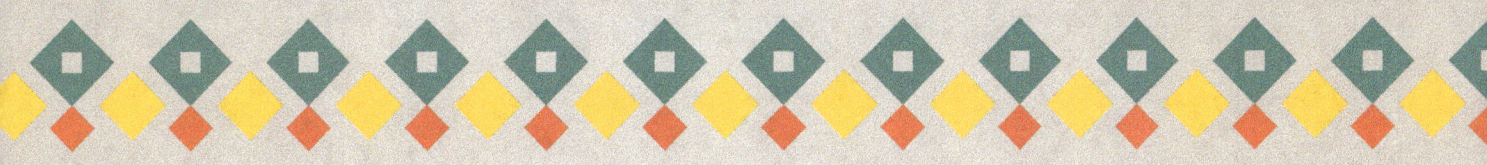

PARTS MAPPING

Close your eyes and imagine that you are landing inside of yourself, where you can clearly feel the presence of your parts.

What do you notice?

Is there a part that feels most present or alive? Using the prompts below, draw and journal your responses below on the following pages.

1. **Part's Name**
2. **Part's Purpose/Role**
3. **Part's Emotion/Feeling/Thoughts**
4. **Somatic Location of Part**
5. **Part's fears, anxieties, or concerns**
6. **Part's Characteristics (i.e., color, shape, size, sound, age, energy)**
7. **What do you need each part to know about you?**
8. **Is the part a protector (i.e., manager or firefighter) or an exile?**
9. **What else does the part need you to know about it?**

PARTS MAPPING SPACE

PARTS MAPPING SPACE

"Freeing yourself was one thing, claiming ownership of that freed self was another."

~TONI MORRISON

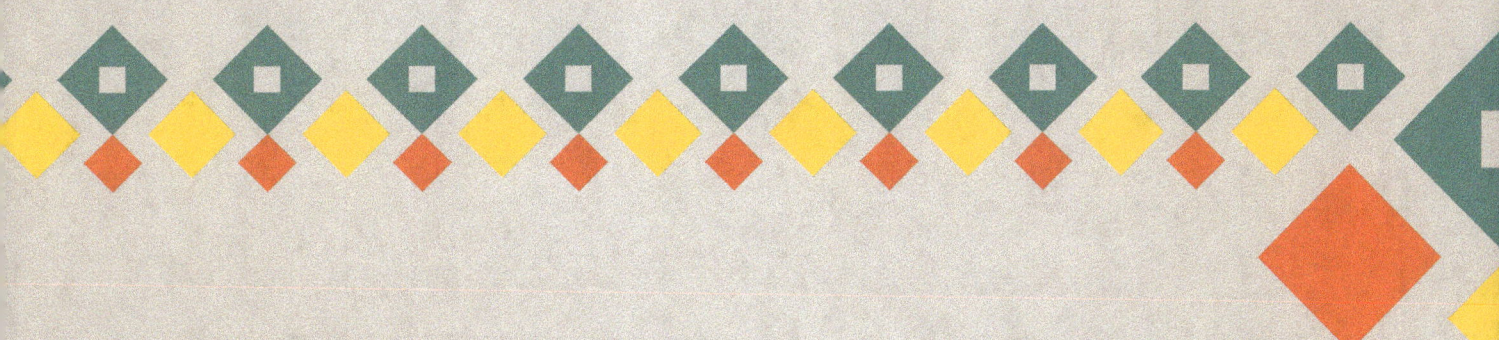

RITUALS

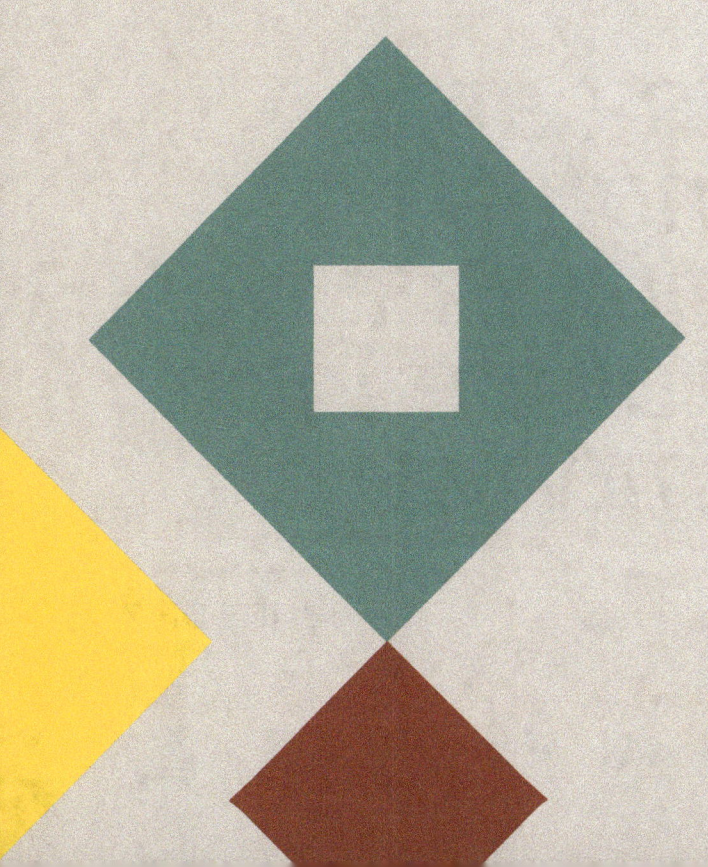

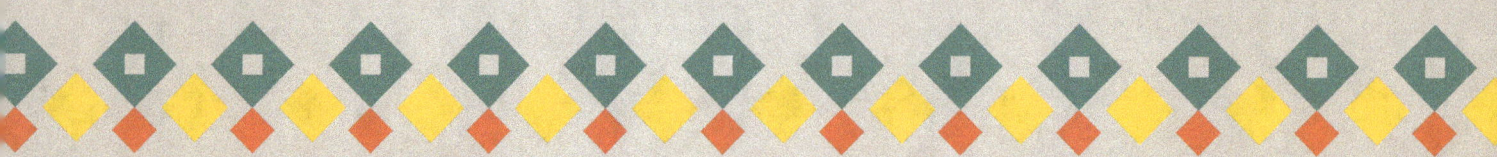

"Rituals carry meaningful intentions that turn your life into a ceremony."

~JULIET DIAZ

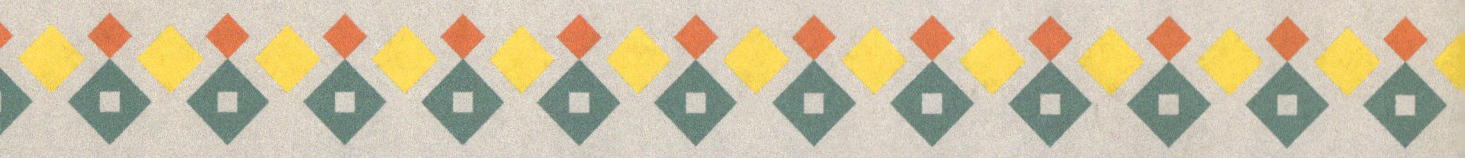

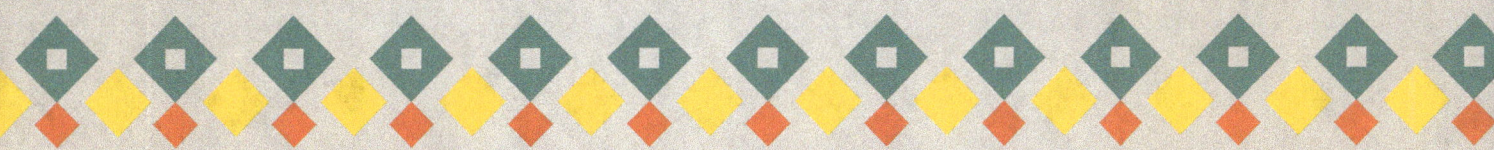

What rituals are important to you and will be a part of this journey?

1. Spending time with your Exile
2. Practice acknowledging your activated parts
3. Limiting social media and screen time
4. Spending time in nature
5. Daily journaling
6. Practicing gratitude
7. Reading
8. Committing to a bedtime routine
9. Meditating
10. Massage/Facial
11. Rest
12. Hygiene
13. Inner Child/ Exile Altar
14. Ancestral Altar
15. Exercise
16. Prayer
17. Somatic Bodywork
18. Cooking/Baking
19. Dancing/Singing
20. Painting/Drawing/Creating/Sculpting
21. Nature/Forest Bathing/Sunbathing/Hiking
22. Connecting with safe friends/community
23. Attending integration circles
24. Spending time with spiritual leaders/mentors
25. Connecting with psychedelic-trained or psychedelic-affirming mental health providers
26. _____
27. _____
28. _____
29. _____
30. _____

"I believe the wound is also the place where the skin reencounters itself, asking of each end, where have you been?"

~OCEAN VUONG

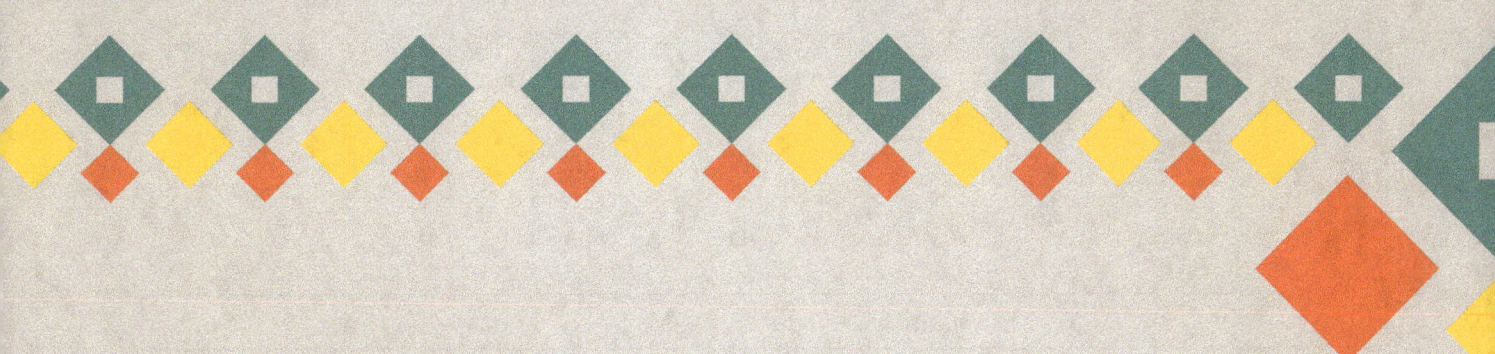

MICRODOSE TRACKERS

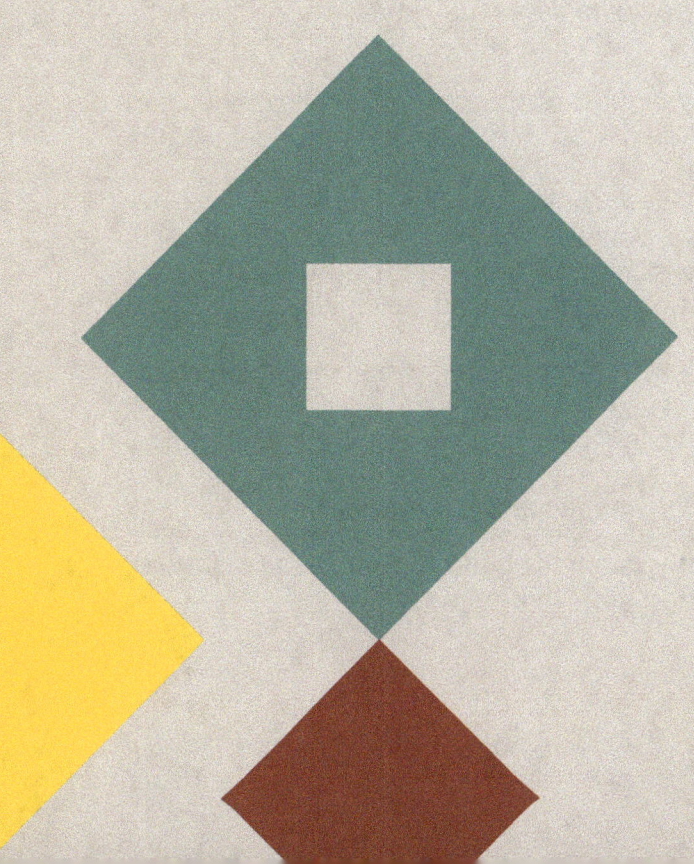

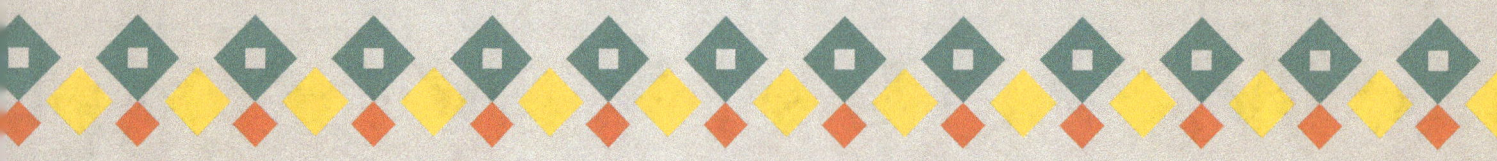

4 WEEK MICRODOSING TRACKER

Week	Sun	Mon	Tue	Wed	Thurs	Fri	Sat
1							
2							
3							
4							

PART'S INTENTIONS:
_____
_____

SELF-ENERGY INTENTIONS:
_____
_____

Have you noticed any shifts in your ability to navigate day-to-day stressors, discomfort, or triggers?

- Have you noticed any changes in how you process trauma or painful experiences?
- How are you feeling about your identity (i.e., race, gender, or sexual orientation)?
- How often are you feeling guilt or shame?
- Have you noticed any changes in how you relate to friends and family?
- How comfortable are you with expressing yourself in private and public spaces?
- Has microdosing impacted how you address boundaries, consent, pleasure, or intimacy?
- How connected do you feel to a higher power, nature, God, spirituality, or personal beliefs?
- Have you noticed any shifts in your body as they relate to tension, pain, numbness, or dissociation?
- Have you experienced any improvements in movement, creativity, communication, or cultural expression?
- Have you felt more connected to your purpose, ancestry, or power?

Note: Tracking these questions consistently can help build a clear picture of how microdosing may (or may not) be supporting your overall well-being.

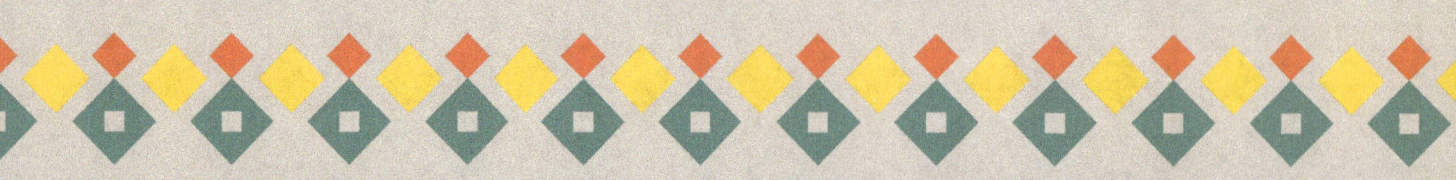

JOURNALING PAGE

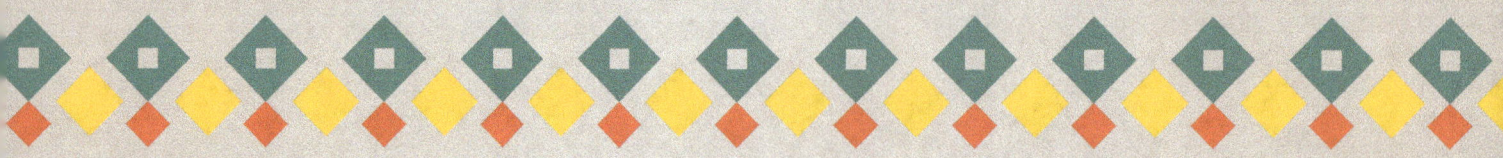

4 WEEK MICRODOSING TRACKER

Week	Sun	Mon	Tue	Wed	Thurs	Fri	Sat
1							
2							
3							
4							

PART'S INTENTIONS:

_____

_____

SELF-ENERGY INTENTIONS:

_____

_____

Have you noticed any shifts in your ability to navigate day-to-day stressors, discomfort, or triggers?

- Have you noticed any changes in how you process trauma or painful experiences?
- How are you feeling about your identity (i.e., race, gender, or sexual orientation)?
- How often are you feeling guilt or shame?
- Have you noticed any changes in how you relate to friends and family?
- How comfortable are you with expressing yourself in private and public spaces?
- Has microdosing impacted how you address boundaries, consent, pleasure, or intimacy?
- How connected do you feel to a higher power, nature, God, spirituality, or personal beliefs?
- Have you noticed any shifts in your body as they relate to tension, pain, numbness, or dissociation?
- Have you experienced any improvements in movement, creativity, communication, or cultural expression?
- Have you felt more connected to your purpose, ancestry, or power?

Note: Tracking these questions consistently can help build a clear picture of how microdosing may (or may not) be supporting your overall well-being.

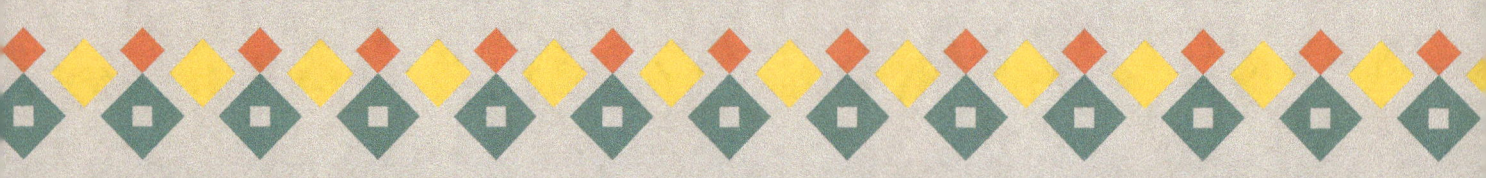

JOURNALING PAGE

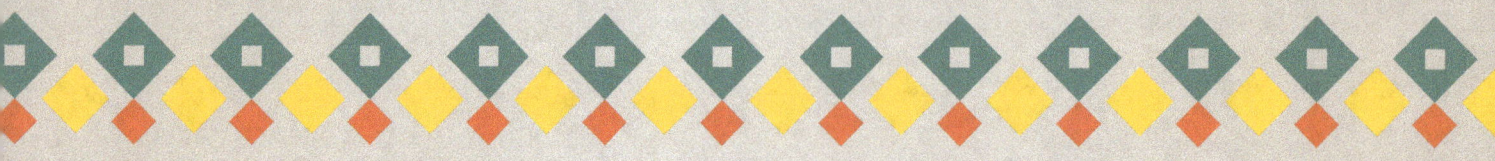

4 WEEK MICRODOSING TRACKER

Week	Sun	Mon	Tue	Wed	Thurs	Fri	Sat
1							
2							
3							
4							

PART'S INTENTIONS:
_____
_____

SELF-ENERGY INTENTIONS:
_____
_____

Have you noticed any shifts in your ability to navigate day-to-day stressors, discomfort, or triggers?

- Have you noticed any changes in how you process trauma or painful experiences?
- How are you feeling about your identity (i.e., race, gender, or sexual orientation)?
- How often are you feeling guilt or shame?
- Have you noticed any changes in how you relate to friends and family?
- How comfortable are you with expressing yourself in private and public spaces?
- Has microdosing impacted how you address boundaries, consent, pleasure, or intimacy?
- How connected do you feel to a higher power, nature, God, spirituality, or personal beliefs?
- Have you noticed any shifts in your body as they relate to tension, pain, numbness, or dissociation?
- Have you experienced any improvements in movement, creativity, communication, or cultural expression?
- Have you felt more connected to your purpose, ancestry, or power?

Note: Tracking these questions consistently can help build a clear picture of how microdosing may (or may not) be supporting your overall well-being.

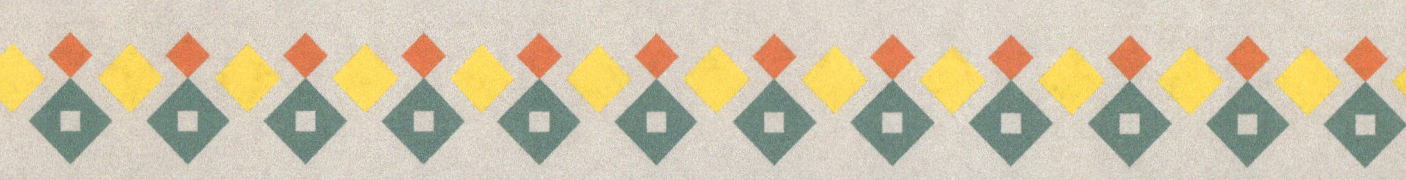

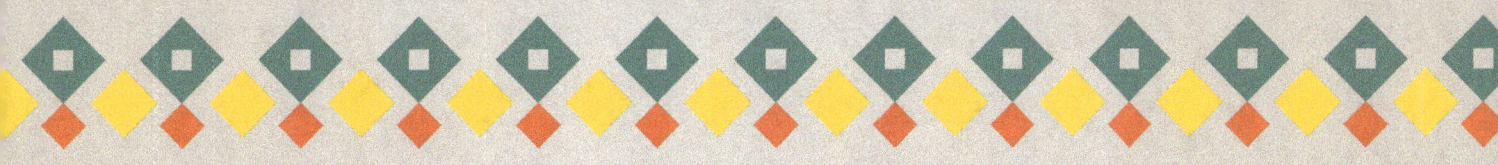

JOURNALING PAGE

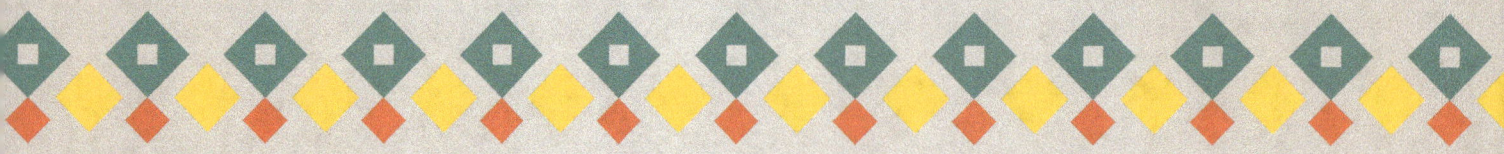

4 WEEK MICRODOSING TRACKER

Week	Sun	Mon	Tue	Wed	Thurs	Fri	Sat
1							
2							
3							
4							

PART'S INTENTIONS:
_____
_____

SELF-ENERGY INTENTIONS:
_____
_____

Have you noticed any shifts in your ability to navigate day-to-day stressors, discomfort, or triggers?

- Have you noticed any changes in how you process trauma or painful experiences?
- How are you feeling about your identity (i.e., race, gender, or sexual orientation)?
- How often are you feeling guilt or shame?
- Have you noticed any changes in how you relate to friends and family?
- How comfortable are you with expressing yourself in private and public spaces?
- Has microdosing impacted how you address boundaries, consent, pleasure, or intimacy?
- How connected do you feel to a higher power, nature, God, spirituality, or personal beliefs?
- Have you noticed any shifts in your body as they relate to tension, pain, numbness, or dissociation?
- Have you experienced any improvements in movement, creativity, communication, or cultural expression?
- Have you felt more connected to your purpose, ancestry, or power?

Note: Tracking these questions consistently can help build a clear picture of how microdosing may (or may not) be supporting your overall well-being.

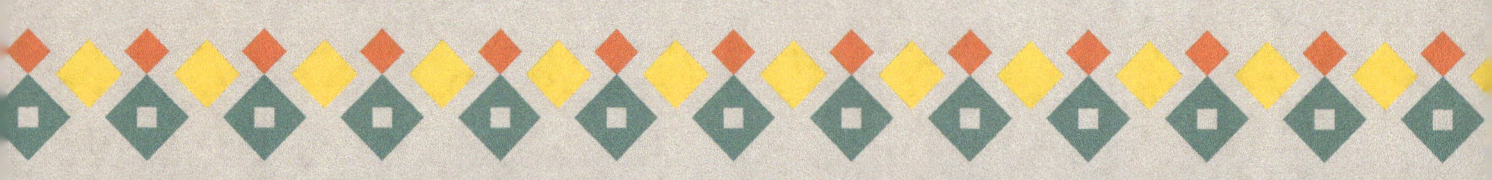

JOURNALING PAGE

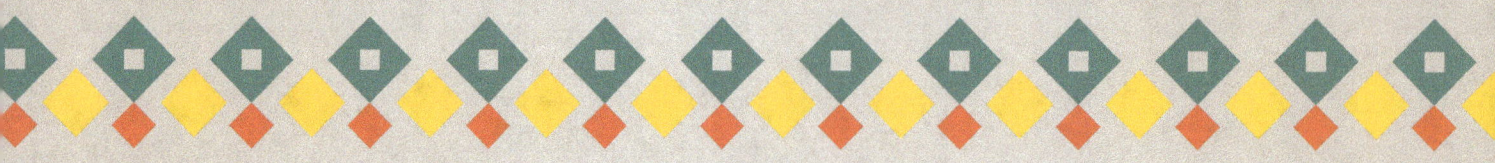

4 WEEK MICRODOSING TRACKER

Week	Sun	Mon	Tue	Wed	Thurs	Fri	Sat
1							
2							
3							
4							

PART'S INTENTIONS:

_____

_____

SELF-ENERGY INTENTIONS:

_____

_____

Have you noticed any shifts in your ability to navigate day-to-day stressors, discomfort, or triggers?

- Have you noticed any changes in how you process trauma or painful experiences?
- How are you feeling about your identity (i.e., race, gender, or sexual orientation)?
- How often are you feeling guilt or shame?
- Have you noticed any changes in how you relate to friends and family?
- How comfortable are you with expressing yourself in private and public spaces?
- Has microdosing impacted how you address boundaries, consent, pleasure, or intimacy?
- How connected do you feel to a higher power, nature, God, spirituality, or personal beliefs?
- Have you noticed any shifts in your body as they relate to tension, pain, numbness, or dissociation?
- Have you experienced any improvements in movement, creativity, communication, or cultural expression?
- Have you felt more connected to your purpose, ancestry, or power?

Note: Tracking these questions consistently can help build a clear picture of how microdosing may (or may not) be supporting your overall well-being.

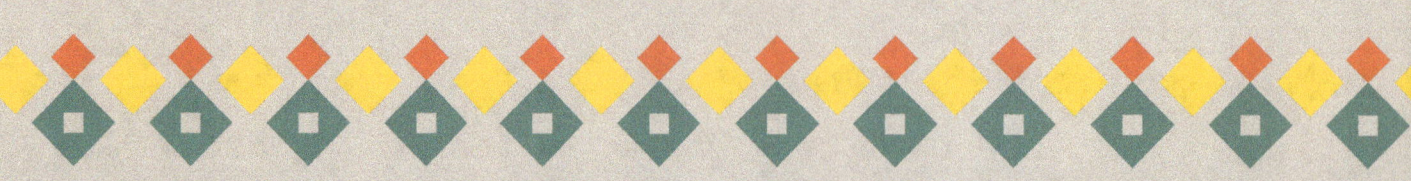

JOURNALING PAGE

_____
_____
_____
_____
_____
_____
_____
_____
_____
_____
_____
_____
_____
_____
_____
_____
_____
_____
_____
_____

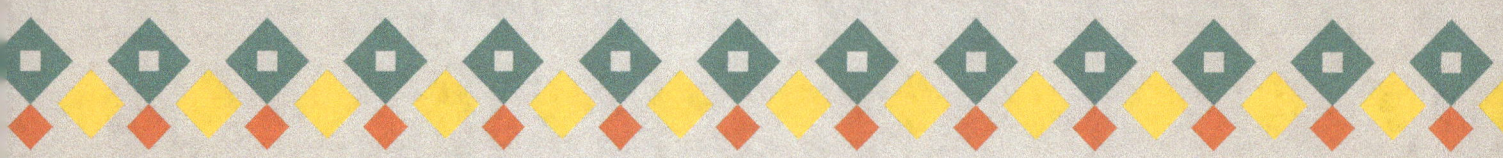

4 WEEK MICRODOSING TRACKER

Week	Sun	Mon	Tue	Wed	Thurs	Fri	Sat
1							
2							
3							
4							

PART'S INTENTIONS:

_____

_____

SELF-ENERGY INTENTIONS:

_____

_____

Have you noticed any shifts in your ability to navigate day-to-day stressors, discomfort, or triggers?

- Have you noticed any changes in how you process trauma or painful experiences?
- How are you feeling about your identity (i.e., race, gender, or sexual orientation)?
- How often are you feeling guilt or shame?
- Have you noticed any changes in how you relate to friends and family?
- How comfortable are you with expressing yourself in private and public spaces?
- Has microdosing impacted how you address boundaries, consent, pleasure, or intimacy?
- How connected do you feel to a higher power, nature, God, spirituality, or personal beliefs?
- Have you noticed any shifts in your body as they relate to tension, pain, numbness, or dissociation?
- Have you experienced any improvements in movement, creativity, communication, or cultural expression?
- Have you felt more connected to your purpose, ancestry, or power?

Note: Tracking these questions consistently can help build a clear picture of how microdosing may (or may not) be supporting your overall well-being.

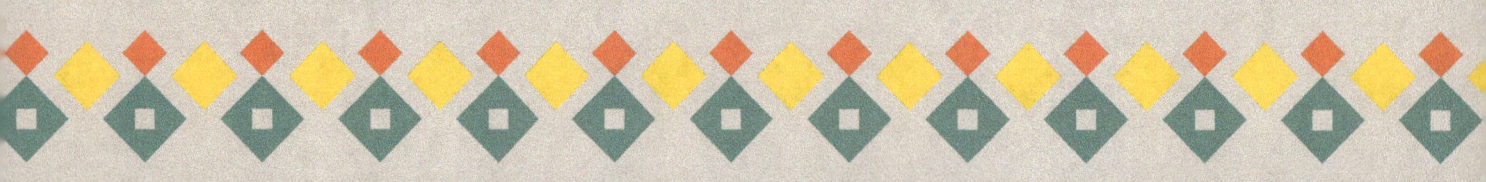

JOURNALING PAGE

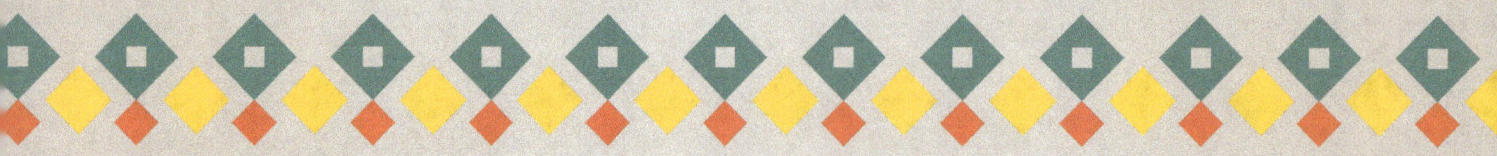

4 WEEK MICRODOSING TRACKER

Week	Sun	Mon	Tue	Wed	Thurs	Fri	Sat
1							
2							
3							
4							

PART'S INTENTIONS:
_____
_____

SELF-ENERGY INTENTIONS:
_____
_____

Have you noticed any shifts in your ability to navigate day-to-day stressors, discomfort, or triggers?

- Have you noticed any changes in how you process trauma or painful experiences?
- How are you feeling about your identity (i.e., race, gender, or sexual orientation)?
- How often are you feeling guilt or shame?
- Have you noticed any changes in how you relate to friends and family?
- How comfortable are you with expressing yourself in private and public spaces?
- Has microdosing impacted how you address boundaries, consent, pleasure, or intimacy?
- How connected do you feel to a higher power, nature, God, spirituality, or personal beliefs?
- Have you noticed any shifts in your body as they relate to tension, pain, numbness, or dissociation?
- Have you experienced any improvements in movement, creativity, communication, or cultural expression?
- Have you felt more connected to your purpose, ancestry, or power?

Note: Tracking these questions consistently can help build a clear picture of how microdosing may (or may not) be supporting your overall well-being.

LIBERATION

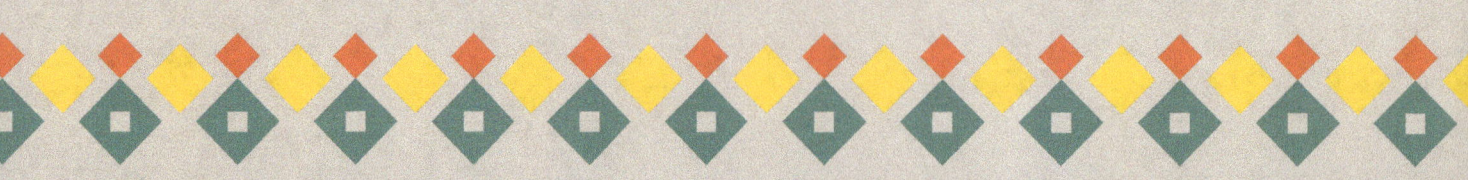

JOURNALING PAGE

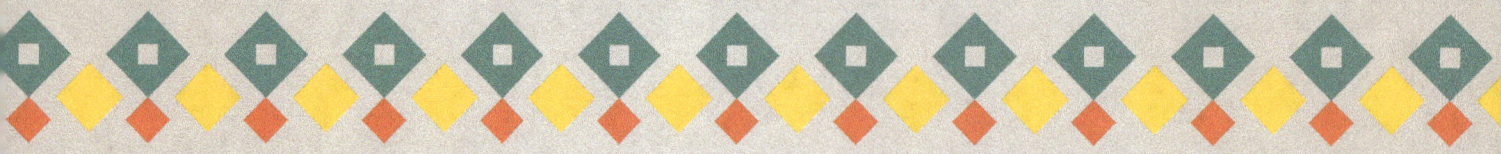

4 WEEK MICRODOSING TRACKER

Week	Sun	Mon	Tue	Wed	Thurs	Fri	Sat
1							
2							
3							
4							

PART'S INTENTIONS:
_____
_____

SELF-ENERGY INTENTIONS:
_____
_____

Have you noticed any shifts in your ability to navigate day-to-day stressors, discomfort, or triggers?

- Have you noticed any changes in how you process trauma or painful experiences?
- How are you feeling about your identity (i.e., race, gender, or sexual orientation)?
- How often are you feeling guilt or shame?
- Have you noticed any changes in how you relate to friends and family?
- How comfortable are you with expressing yourself in private and public spaces?
- Has microdosing impacted how you address boundaries, consent, pleasure, or intimacy?
- How connected do you feel to a higher power, nature, God, spirituality, or personal beliefs?
- Have you noticed any shifts in your body as they relate to tension, pain, numbness, or dissociation?
- Have you experienced any improvements in movement, creativity, communication, or cultural expression?
- Have you felt more connected to your purpose, ancestry, or power?

Note: Tracking these questions consistently can help build a clear picture of how microdosing may (or may not) be supporting your overall well-being.

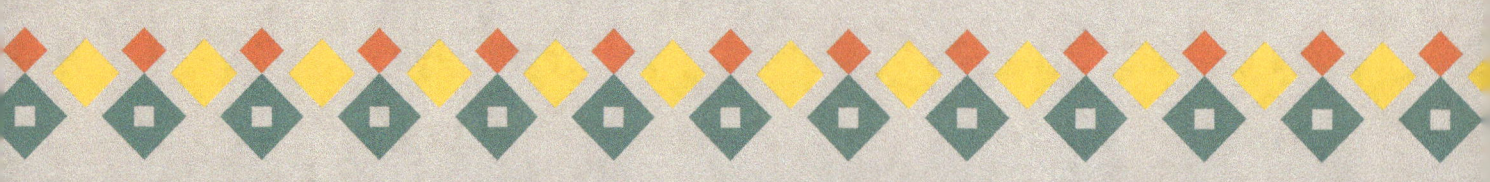

JOURNALING PAGE

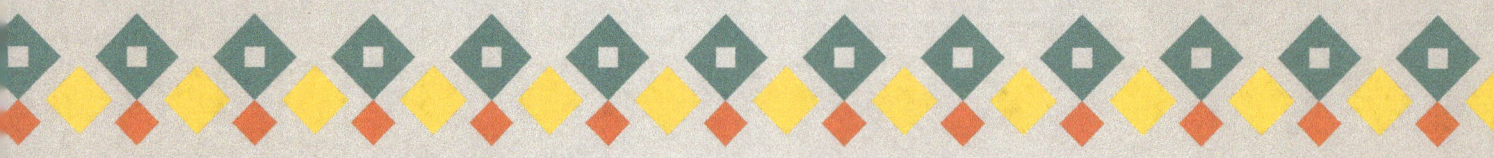

4 WEEK MICRODOSING TRACKER

Week	Sun	Mon	Tue	Wed	Thurs	Fri	Sat
1							
2							
3							
4							

PART'S INTENTIONS:
_____
_____

SELF-ENERGY INTENTIONS:
_____
_____

Have you noticed any shifts in your ability to navigate day-to-day stressors, discomfort, or triggers?

- Have you noticed any changes in how you process trauma or painful experiences?
- How are you feeling about your identity (i.e., race, gender, or sexual orientation)?
- How often are you feeling guilt or shame?
- Have you noticed any changes in how you relate to friends and family?
- How comfortable are you with expressing yourself in private and public spaces?
- Has microdosing impacted how you address boundaries, consent, pleasure, or intimacy?
- How connected do you feel to a higher power, nature, God, spirituality, or personal beliefs?
- Have you noticed any shifts in your body as they relate to tension, pain, numbness, or dissociation?
- Have you experienced any improvements in movement, creativity, communication, or cultural expression?
- Have you felt more connected to your purpose, ancestry, or power?

Note: Tracking these questions consistently can help build a clear picture of how microdosing may (or may not) be supporting your overall well-being.

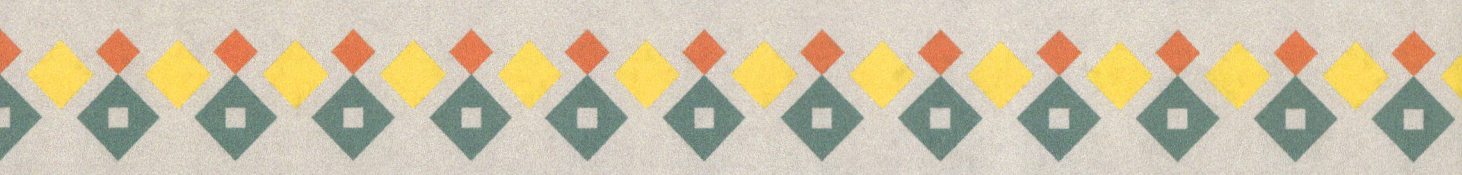

JOURNALING PAGE

_____
_____
_____
_____
_____
_____
_____
_____
_____
_____
_____
_____
_____
_____
_____
_____
_____
_____
_____
_____

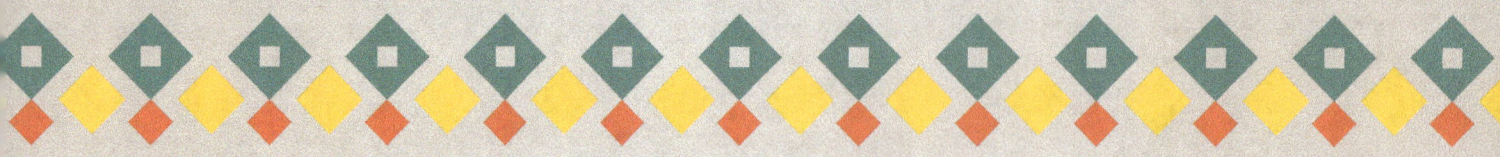

4 WEEK MICRODOSING TRACKER

Week	Sun	Mon	Tue	Wed	Thurs	Fri	Sat
1							
2							
3							
4							

PART'S INTENTIONS:

_____

_____

SELF-ENERGY INTENTIONS:

_____

_____

Have you noticed any shifts in your ability to navigate day-to-day stressors, discomfort, or triggers?

- Have you noticed any changes in how you process trauma or painful experiences?
- How are you feeling about your identity (i.e., race, gender, or sexual orientation)?
- How often are you feeling guilt or shame?
- Have you noticed any changes in how you relate to friends and family?
- How comfortable are you with expressing yourself in private and public spaces?
- Has microdosing impacted how you address boundaries, consent, pleasure, or intimacy?
- How connected do you feel to a higher power, nature, God, spirituality, or personal beliefs?
- Have you noticed any shifts in your body as they relate to tension, pain, numbness, or dissociation?
- Have you experienced any improvements in movement, creativity, communication, or cultural expression?
- Have you felt more connected to your purpose, ancestry, or power?

Note: Tracking these questions consistently can help build a clear picture of how microdosing may (or may not) be supporting your overall well-being.

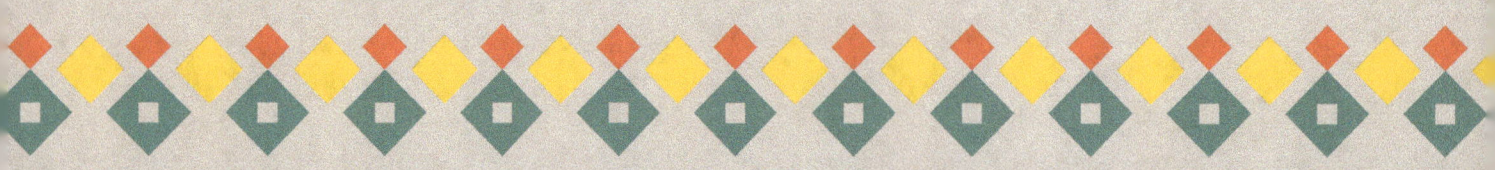

JOURNALING PAGE

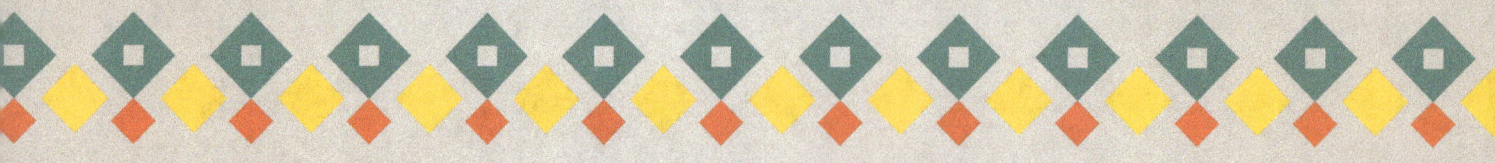

4 WEEK MICRODOSING TRACKER

Week	Sun	Mon	Tue	Wed	Thurs	Fri	Sat
1							
2							
3							
4							

PART'S INTENTIONS:

_____

_____

SELF-ENERGY INTENTIONS:

_____

_____

Have you noticed any shifts in your ability to navigate day-to-day stressors, discomfort, or triggers?

- Have you noticed any changes in how you process trauma or painful experiences?
- How are you feeling about your identity (i.e., race, gender, or sexual orientation)?
- How often are you feeling guilt or shame?
- Have you noticed any changes in how you relate to friends and family?
- How comfortable are you with expressing yourself in private and public spaces?
- Has microdosing impacted how you address boundaries, consent, pleasure, or intimacy?
- How connected do you feel to a higher power, nature, God, spirituality, or personal beliefs?
- Have you noticed any shifts in your body as they relate to tension, pain, numbness, or dissociation?
- Have you experienced any improvements in movement, creativity, communication, or cultural expression?
- Have you felt more connected to your purpose, ancestry, or power?

Note: Tracking these questions consistently can help build a clear picture of how microdosing may (or may not) be supporting your overall well-being.

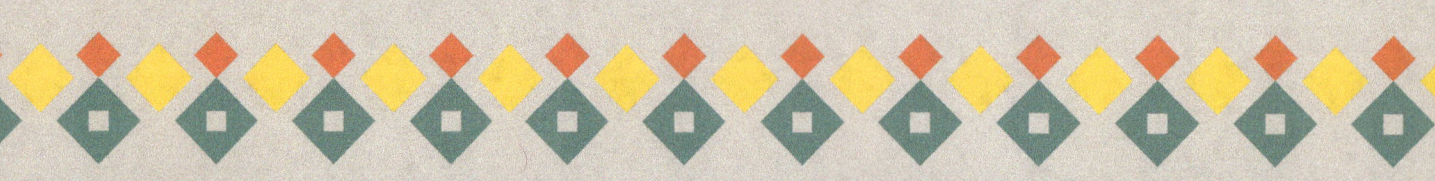

JOURNALING PAGE

_____
_____
_____
_____
_____
_____
_____
_____
_____
_____
_____
_____
_____
_____
_____
_____
_____
_____
_____

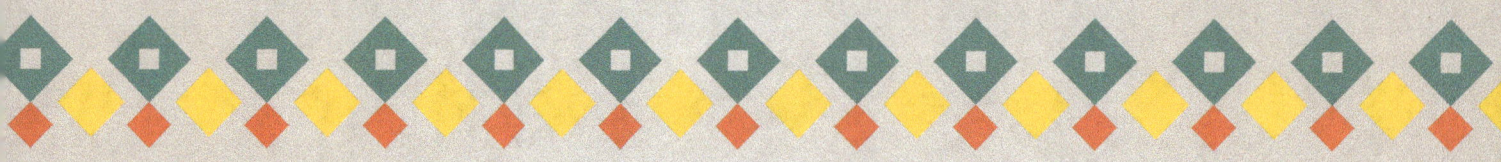

4 WEEK MICRODOSING TRACKER

Week	Sun	Mon	Tue	Wed	Thurs	Fri	Sat
1							
2							
3							
4							

PART'S INTENTIONS:
_____
_____

SELF-ENERGY INTENTIONS:
_____
_____

Have you noticed any shifts in your ability to navigate day-to-day stressors, discomfort, or triggers?

- Have you noticed any changes in how you process trauma or painful experiences?
- How are you feeling about your identity (i.e., race, gender, or sexual orientation)?
- How often are you feeling guilt or shame?
- Have you noticed any changes in how you relate to friends and family?
- How comfortable are you with expressing yourself in private and public spaces?
- Has microdosing impacted how you address boundaries, consent, pleasure, or intimacy?
- How connected do you feel to a higher power, nature, God, spirituality, or personal beliefs?
- Have you noticed any shifts in your body as they relate to tension, pain, numbness, or dissociation?
- Have you experienced any improvements in movement, creativity, communication, or cultural expression?
- Have you felt more connected to your purpose, ancestry, or power?

Note: Tracking these questions consistently can help build a clear picture of how microdosing may (or may not) be supporting your overall well-being.

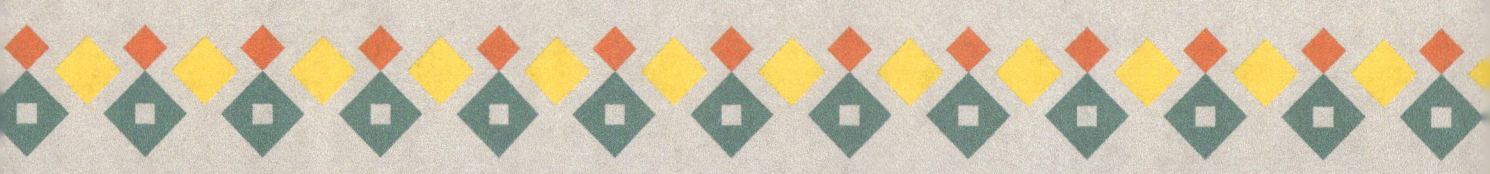

JOURNALING PAGE

_____
_____
_____
_____
_____
_____
_____
_____
_____
_____
_____
_____
_____
_____
_____
_____
_____
_____
_____
_____

"I now understand that life, and living it, is more about being present. I'm now aware that the not-so-happy memories lie in wait; but the hope and the joy also lie in wait."

~VIOLA DAVIS

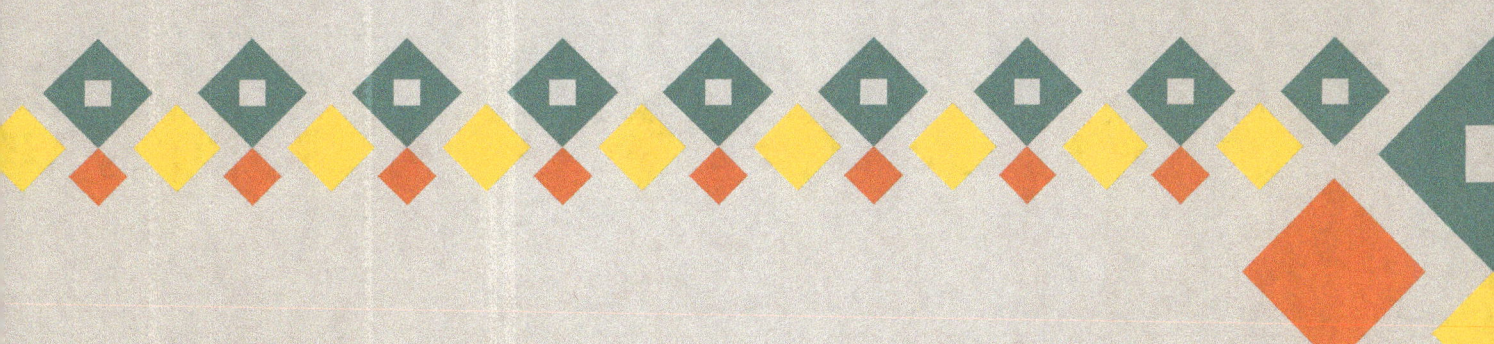

SELF-ENERGY ASSESSMENTS

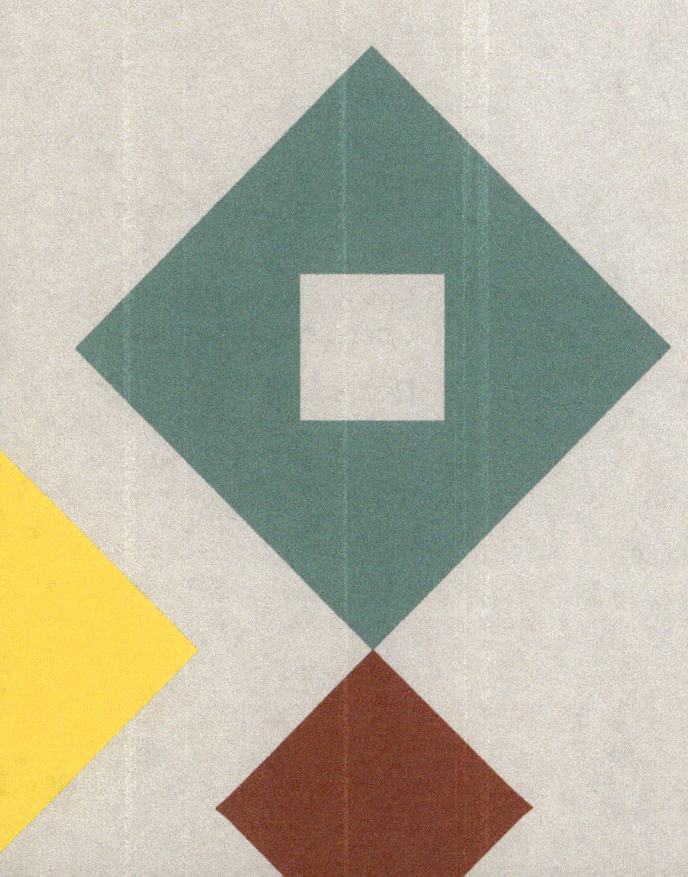

SELF-ENERGY ASSESSMENT #1

Check the box next to the timeframe during which self-energy is being monitored.

- ☐ Before the medicine experience
- ☐ 24-48 hours after the medicine experience
- ☐ 60 days after the medicine experience

How difficult is it to feel/express/experience the following (on a scale of 1-5 with 5 being the most challenging/difficult):

___ Curiosity

___ Compassion

___ Courage

___ Clarity

___ Calmness

___ Creativity

___ Confidence

___ Connection

___ Pleasure

___ Protection

___ Cultural Expression (i.e., language, traditions, style, movement, and spirituality)

___ Choice

___ Community/Co-creation

___ Comedy/Laughter

___ Celebration

___ Community Care

___ Ceremony

___ Consent

___ Contentment

___ Continuity

___ Tenderness

___ Unity

___ Speaking up

___ Social Justice

___ Hope

___ Joy

___ Self-Forgiveness/Grace

___ Boundaries

___ Anger

___ Intuition

___ Feminine Erotic Power/Passion

___ Emancipation of Oppressive Systems

___ Reciprocity

___ Respect for animals/nature/people

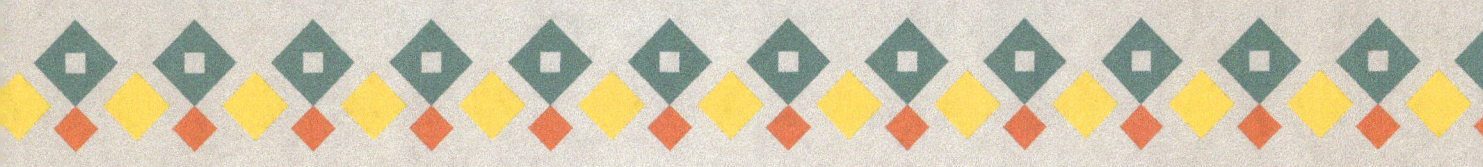

SELF-ENERGY ASSESSMENT #2

Check the box next to the timeframe during which self-energy is being monitored.

☐ Before the medicine experience
☐ 24-48 hours after the medicine experience
☐ 60 days after the medicine experience

How difficult is it to feel/express/experience the following (on a scale of 1-5 with 5 being the most challenging/difficult):

___ Curiosity

___ Compassion

___ Courage

___ Clarity

___ Calmness

___ Creativity

___ Confidence

___ Connection

___ Pleasure

___ Protection

___ Cultural Expression (i.e., language, traditions, style, movement, and spirituality)

___ Choice

___ Community/Co-creation

___ Comedy/Laughter

___ Celebration

___ Community Care

___ Ceremony

___ Consent

___ Contentment

___ Continuity

___ Tenderness

___ Unity

___ Speaking up

___ Social Justice

___ Hope

___ Joy

___ Self-Forgiveness/Grace

___ Boundaries

___ Anger

___ Intuition

___ Feminine Erotic Power/Passion

___ Emancipation of Oppressive Systems

___ Reciprocity

___ Respect for animals/nature/people

SELF-ENERGY ASSESSMENT #3

Check the box next to the timeframe during which self-energy is being monitored.

☐ Before the medicine experience
☐ 24-48 hours after the medicine experience
☐ 60 days after the medicine experience

How difficult is it to feel/express/experience the following (on a scale of 1-5 with 5 being the most challenging/difficult):

___ Curiosity

___ Compassion

___ Courage

___ Clarity

___ Calmness

___ Creativity

___ Confidence

___ Connection

___ Pleasure

___ Protection

___ Cultural Expression (i.e., language, traditions, style, movement, and spirituality)

___ Choice

___ Community/Co-creation

___ Comedy/Laughter

___ Celebration

___ Community Care

___ Ceremony

___ Consent

___ Contentment

___ Continuity

___ Tenderness

___ Unity

___ Speaking up

___ Social Justice

___ Hope

___ Joy

___ Self-Forgiveness/Grace

___ Boundaries

___ Anger

___ Intuition

___ Feminine Erotic Power/Passion

___ Emancipation of Oppressive Systems

___ Reciprocity

___ Respect for animals/nature/people

LIBERATION

JOURNALING PAGE

"To survive,
Let the past
Teach you--
Past customs,
Struggles,
Leaders and thinkers.
Let
These
Help you.
Let them inspire you,
Warn you,
Give you strength.
But beware:
God is Change.
Past is past.
What was
Cannot
Come again.

To survive,
know the past.
Let it touch you.
Then let
The past
Go."

~OCTAVIA BUTLER

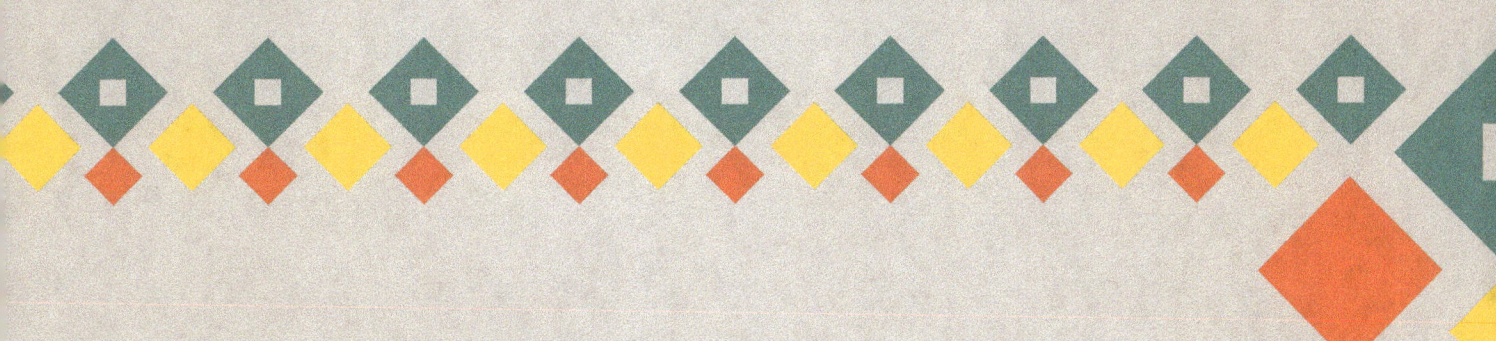

INTEGRATION JOURNAL PROMPTS

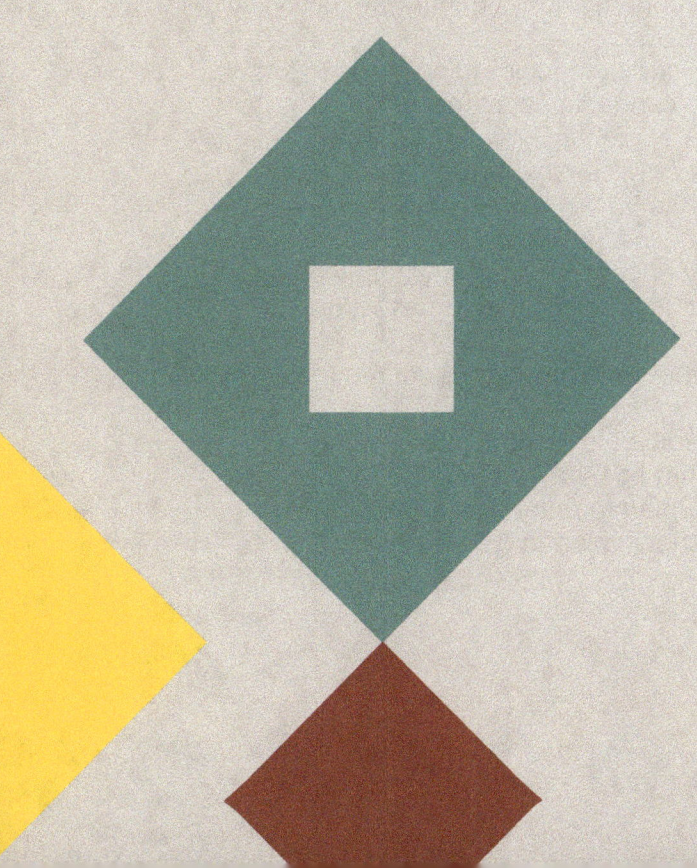

INTEGRATION JOURNAL PROMPTS

1. The portion of my journey that I most want to remember is…
2. If my closest friend asks about the experience, I will share…
3. To deepen my integration experience, I will take the following actions…
4. Since my medicine experience, I have felt…
5. The Self inside of me wants me to remember…
6. To bring more ease or peace into my life, I plan to…
7. Imagining my parts that feel alone, ashamed, or neglected — if they could speak what would they say…?
8. The part of me that holds sadness tries to comfort me by… _
9. The parts of me that most show up in a relationship with others are… _
10. I feel most connected to my self-energy when…
11. The parts that carry legacy burdens about my body, identity, sexuality, societal expectations, or worth want me to know…
12. The parts that feel silenced, invisible, or disempowered want me to know…
13. When I reflect on ancestral or cultural connections, I feel…
14. The parts that hold trauma related to my identity have shown me…
15. I feel unconditional love for myself *and* my parts when…
16. I inherited the following qualities or traits from my ancestors…
17. My ancestors have passed down the following lessons…
18. If I could have a conversation with my ancestors, here is what I would say…
19. I feel love in the following ways, and this is how I plan to pass it on…
20. If my body could speak, it would say…
21. Parts of me are either trying to love, meet a need, or protect me in the following ways…
22. The depth, twists, and turns of my medicine experience were…
23. Healing is my birthright, and this is what I desire to heal…
24. Rest is my birthright, and this is how I plan to rest…
25. Liberation is my birthright, and this is how I plan to get free…

JOURNALING PAGE

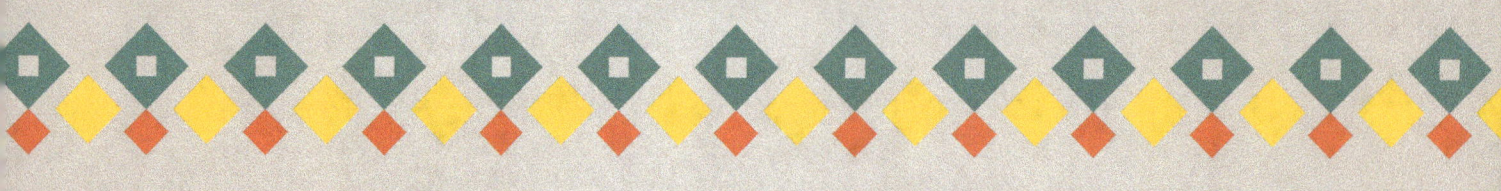

JOURNALING PAGE

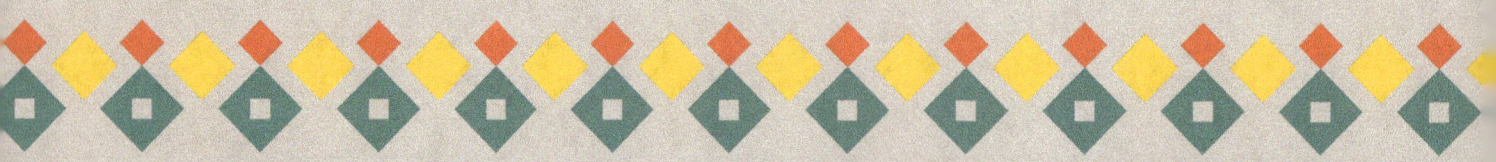

JOURNALING PAGE

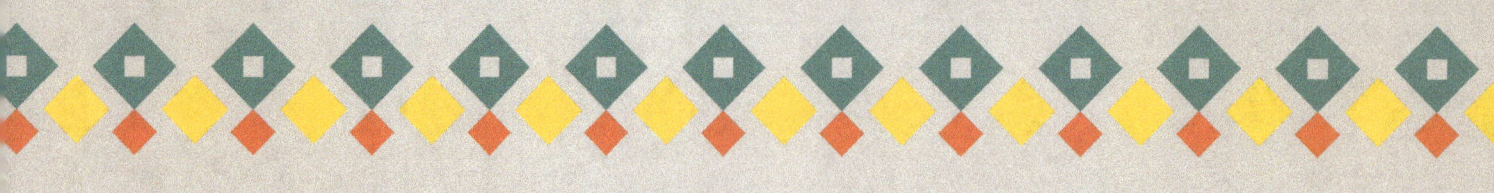

JOURNALING PAGE

_____
_____
_____
_____
_____
_____
_____
_____
_____
_____
_____
_____
_____
_____
_____
_____
_____

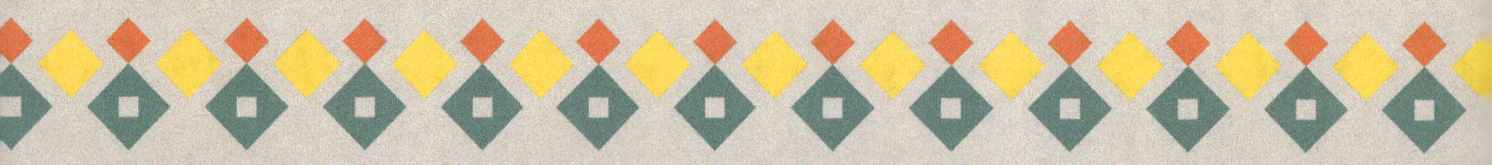

JOURNALING PAGE

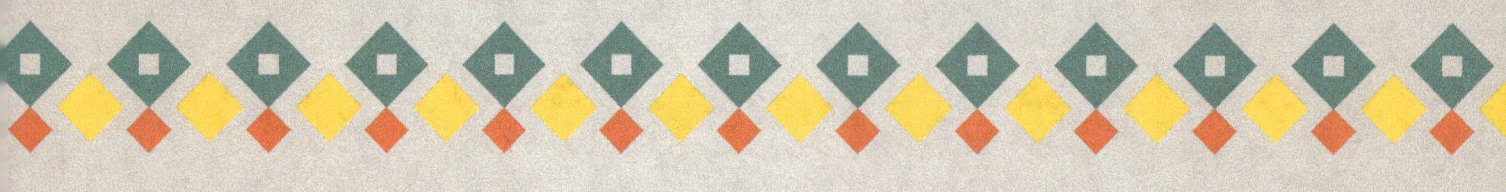

JOURNALING PAGE

_____
_____
_____
_____
_____
_____
_____
_____
_____
_____
_____
_____
_____
_____
_____
_____
_____
_____

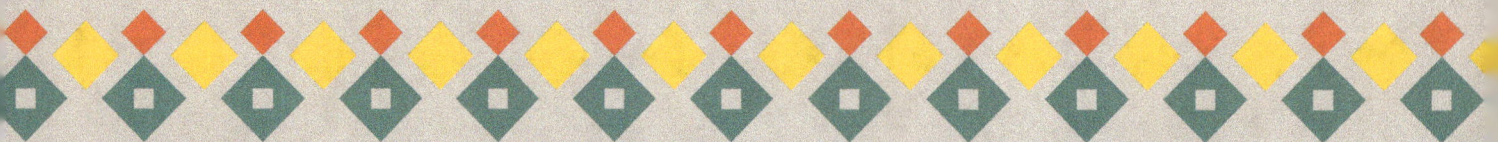

JOURNALING PAGE

GUIDED JOURNALING WORKSHEET

"Simplicity, patience, compassion.

These three are your greatest treasures.

Simple in actions and thoughts, you return to the source of being.

Patient with both friends and enemies,

you accord with the way things are.

Compassionate toward yourself, you reconcile all beings in the world."

~LAO TZU

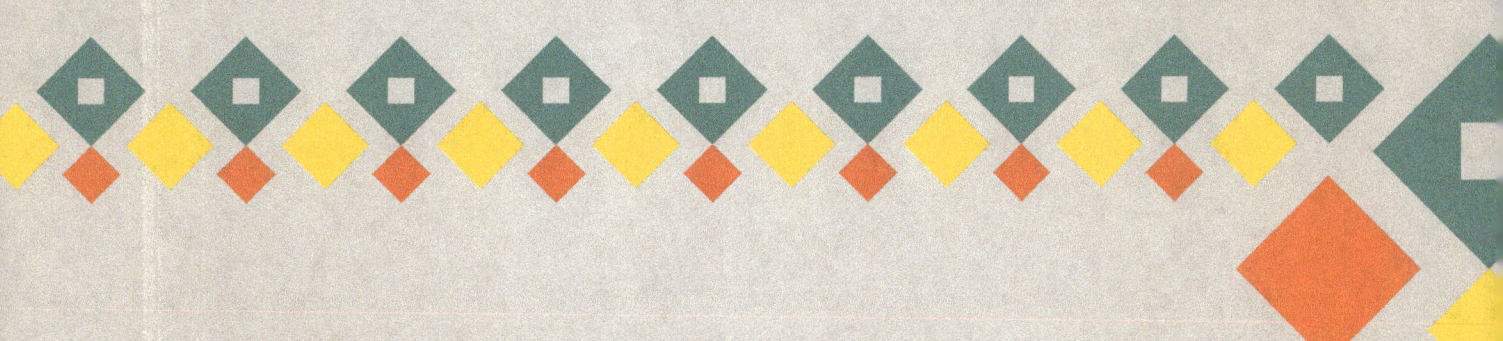

LETTERS

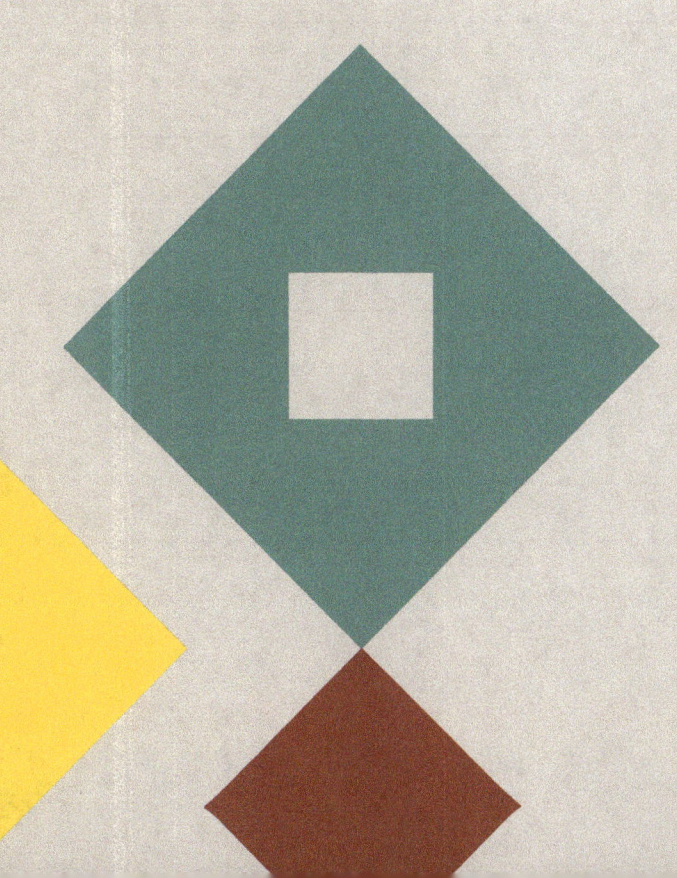

LETTER TO YOUR YOUNGER SELF

Use the space below to write a letter to your younger self— the Exile — that visited you during your medicine journey. You can also use the space below to process anything that your Exile wants you to know about them.

Date: _____

_____
_____
_____
_____
_____
_____
_____
_____
_____
_____
_____
_____
_____
_____
_____
_____

JOURNALING PAGE

LETTER TO YOUR PARTS

Use the space below to write a letter to any part(s) that visited you during your medicine journey. You can also use this space to process anything that your parts want you to know about them.

Date: _____

_____
_____
_____
_____
_____
_____
_____
_____
_____
_____
_____
_____
_____
_____

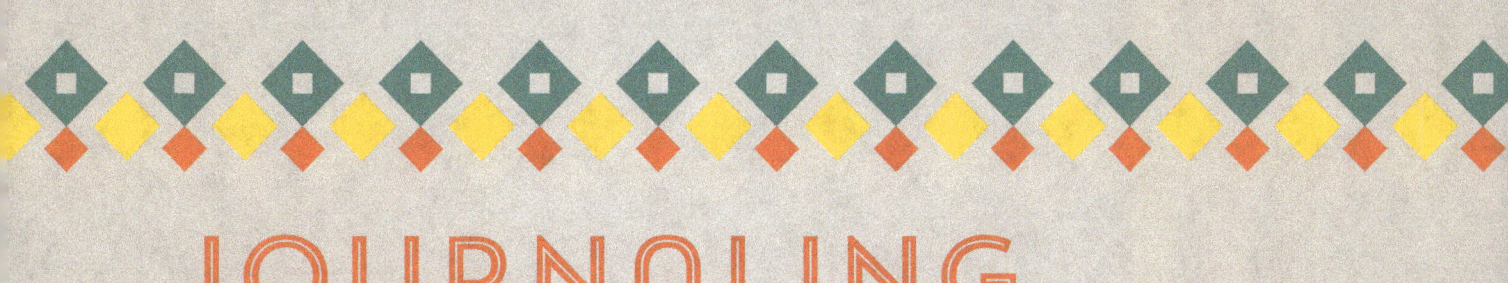

JOURNALING PAGE

_____
_____
_____
_____
_____
_____
_____
_____
_____
_____
_____
_____
_____
_____
_____
_____
_____

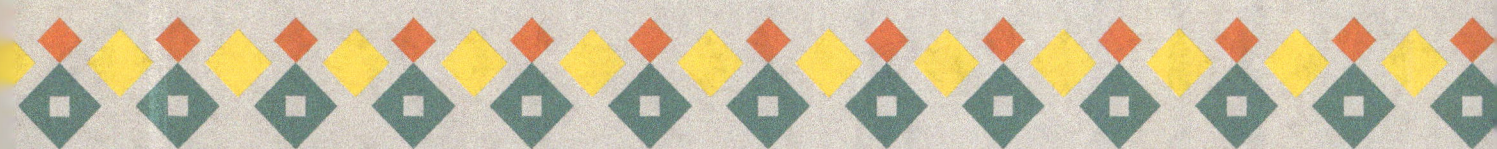

"We deserve to experience love fully, equally, without shame and without compromise."

~ELLIOTT PAGE

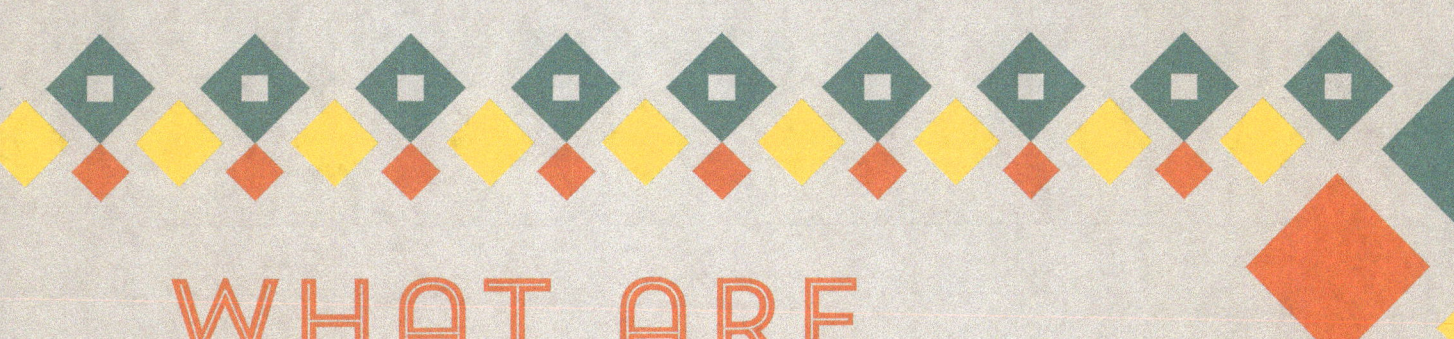

WHAT ARE THE PARTS?

Date: _____

Use this page to identify parts as they show up. Draw or write in the space provided. The purpose is to remember and understand your internal system and how your parts interact with each other to protect you. Parts mapping and tracking are powerful tools to explore themes during post-integration sessions, integration circles, coaching, or therapy sessions.

- **What is the story?**
- **What are the thoughts?**
- **What are the feelings?**
- **What is the behavior or beliefs?**
- **What are the somatic sensations?**
- **What are the dreams/nightmares?**

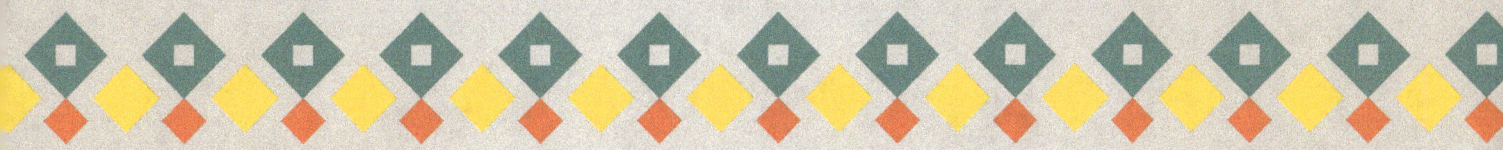

WHAT ARE THE PARTS?

Date: _____

Use this page to identify parts as they show up. Draw or write in the space provided. The purpose is to remember and understand your internal system and how your parts interact with each other to protect you. Parts mapping and tracking are powerful tools to explore themes during post-integration sessions, integration circles, coaching, or therapy sessions.

- **What is the story?**
- **What are the thoughts?**
- **What are the feelings?**
- **What is the behavior or beliefs?**
- **What are the somatic sensations?**
- **What are the dreams/nightmares?**

LIBERATION

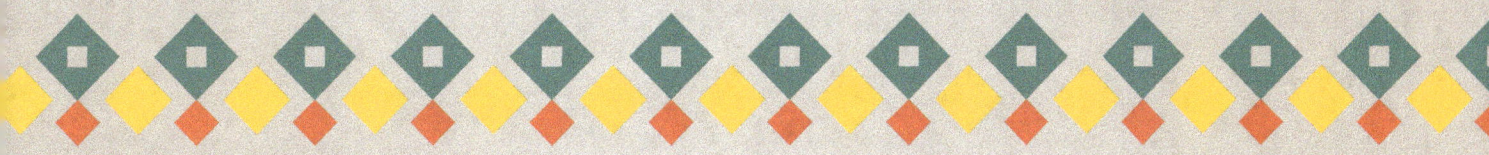

WHAT ARE THE PARTS?

Date: _____

Use this page to identify parts as they show up. Draw or write in the space provided. The purpose is to remember and understand your internal system and how your parts interact with each other to protect you. Parts mapping and tracking are powerful tools to explore themes during post-integration sessions, integration circles, coaching, or therapy sessions.

- **What is the story?**
- **What are the thoughts?**
- **What are the feelings?**
- **What is the behavior or beliefs?**
- **What are the somatic sensations?**
- **What are the dreams/nightmares?**

RESOURCE RECOMMENDATIONS

BOOKS

Alter Within, by Juliet Diaz
Altogether Us, by Jenna Riemersma
body rites, by shena j. young
Decolonizing Trauma Work, by Renee Linklater
Internal Family Systems Therapy, Second Edition, by Richard C. Swartz
Kwanzaa: A Celebration of Family, Community, and Culture, by Maulana Karenga
Post Traumatic Slave Syndrome, by Dr. Joy DeGruy, Ph.D
Practicing Kwanzaa Year Round: Affirmations and Activities Around the Seven Principles, by Gwynelle Dismukes
Queering Psychedelics, by Alex Belser
The Pain We Carry, by Natalie Gutierrez
The Spirit of Intimacy, by Sobunfu Some
Whole Medicine: A Guide to Ethics and Harm-Reduction for Psychedelic Therapy and Plant Medicine Communities, by Rachel Martinez
You Are The Medicine, by Asha Frost

MOBILE APPS

www.calm.com
www.insighttimer.com

PODCASTS

When We Speak Podcast with Tasha Hunter
Deeply Well with Devi Brown
The Psychedelic Therapy Podcast with Laura Northrup
The Homecoming Podcast with Dr. Thema
Brown Girls Don't Do Therapy with Diviya Lewis

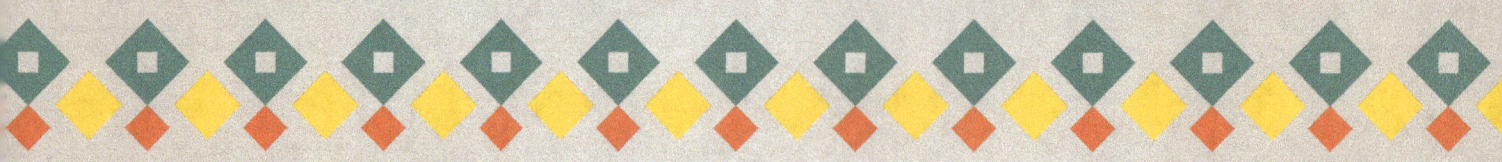

PRACTITIONERS

Alexis Ornellas www.manacounseling.com
Candace Oglesby https://jurneewithcandace.com/
MayRav Nissim www.mayravnissim.com
Nic Wildes, LMHC nicwildes.com
Rebekah Gong www.dearrootedlotus.com

WEBSITES

Finding an IFS Therapist www.selfleadership.org

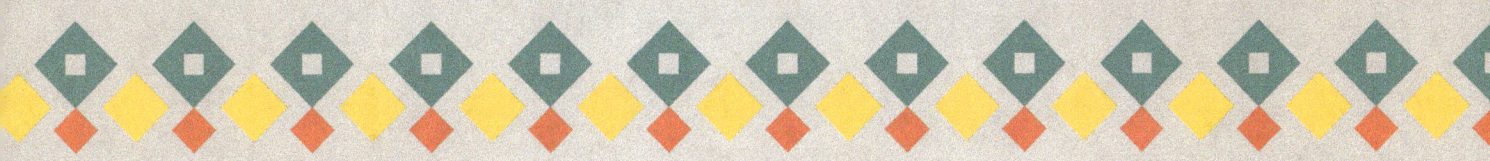

ABOUT THE AUTHOR

FOLLOW ME ON INSTAGRAM AND THREADS @TASHAHUNTERLCSW

Tasha Hunter (she/her/we) is a Black, queer listener, healer, writer, teacher, and advocate. She is a liberation-centered mental health therapist who specializes in working with Black women, femmes, and LGBTQIA+ communities. She believes that healing happens most often when we are seen, heard, and understood by those who value our existence. She also believes that liberation isn't possible without community and collective liberation.

Tasha is a Level 3, certified Internal Family Systems therapist who approaches healing from a non-pathologizing, decolonized lens. She most often provides a safe container for individuals seeking help due to generational trauma, ancestral trauma, inner-child wounding, sexual violence, racism, sexism, oppression, sexual identity/romantic-relationship stressors, and spiritual/religious deconstruction.

Tasha's clinical practice also includes the pre-and-post integration of psychedelic and ancestral medicine experiences, breathwork, somatic practices, spirituality, and ancestral wisdom. She is the author of *tell me where it hurts: poetry, meditations, and divinely-inspired love notes* and her memoir, *What Children Remember*. Her writing has been featured in *She Lives Her Truth* and *please cut up my poems*. She is also the host of the podcast, *When We Speak*. She lives in North Carolina and owns a private mental health practice.

For more information or if you are interested in working with me visit https:// www.tashahunterlcsw.com or email @ tashahunterlcsw@gmail.com. I would love to speak with you about training, workshops, supervision, and consultation.

OTHER BOOKS

If you enjoyed *Liberation*, I invite you to explore my other works. Each book is a reflection of my personal and professional journey. Visit www.tashahunterlcsw.com to find my latest releases and stay connected for future books, events, and more. Let's continue healing together!

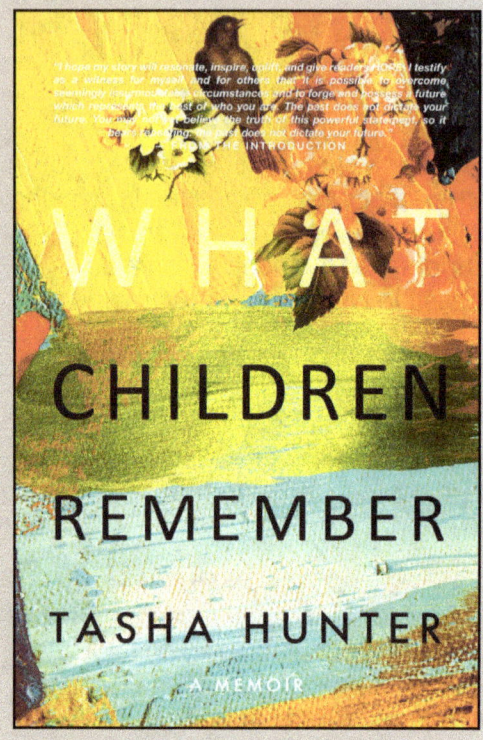
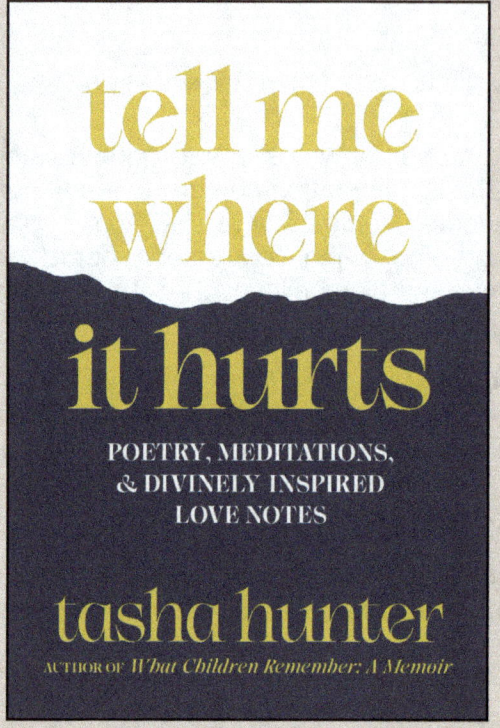

My books are available at Amazon, Books-A-Million, and other major retailers. I encourage you to also support LGBTQIA+ and Global Majority-owned bookstores by purchasing my books through them whenever possible.

HEARTFELT APPRECIATION

A heartfelt thanks to every person who encourages me and continues to support my work. Special thanks to my editor Mellisa, you have been with me since the beginning and our friendship and collaboration means the world. To my family and friends, I love you. To my IFS peers and community, I couldn't have completed this book without you.

Readers, I hope this guide has resonated with you and offered something meaningful for your journey. If you enjoyed it, I would be incredibly grateful if you could take a few moments to leave a review. Your feedback not only helps me as an author, but it also allows others to discover this book and benefit from it as well.

To leave a review, simply visit Amazon/Goodreads and share your thoughts. If you share this or any of my books on social media, tag me on Instagram and Threads @ Tashahunterlcsw.

Thank you again for your support!

www.ingramcontent.com/pod-product-compliance
Lightning Source LLC
Chambersburg PA
CBHW080324080526
44585CB00021B/2455